シンプル
理学療法学
作業療法学
シリーズ

リハビリテーション英語テキスト

English for Students of Rehabilitation

監修
細田多穂
埼玉県立大学名誉教授

編集
飯島博之
埼玉県立大学

濱口豊太
埼玉県立大学

隈元庸夫
埼玉県立大学

南江堂

● 監　修

細田多穂	ほそだ　かずほ	埼玉県立大学名誉教授

● 編　集

飯島博之	いいじま　ひろゆき	埼玉県立大学保健医療福祉学部共通教育科教授
濱口豊太	はまぐち　とよひろ	埼玉県立大学保健医療福祉学部作業療法学科教授
隈元庸夫	くまもと　つねお	北海道千歳リハビリテーション大学健康科学部リハビリテーション学科教授

● 執筆者（執筆順）

飯島博之	いいじま　ひろゆき	埼玉県立大学保健医療福祉学部共通教育科教授
濱口豊太	はまぐち　とよひろ	埼玉県立大学保健医療福祉学部作業療法学科教授
隈元庸夫	くまもと　つねお	北海道千歳リハビリテーション大学健康科学部リハビリテーション学科教授
島崎美登里	しまざき　みどり	埼玉県立大学保健医療福祉学部共通教育科教授
林　幸子	はやし　さちこ	神奈川大学非常勤講師

● 編集協力

橋本康子	はしもと　やすこ	放送大学非常勤講師

監修のことば

　近年，高齢社会を迎え，理学療法士・作業療法士の需要が高まっている．したがって，教育には，これらを目指す学生に対する教育の質を保証し，教育水準の向上および均質化に努める責務がある．

　その一方で学生には，学習した内容を単に"暗記する"だけでなく，"理解して覚える"ということが求められるようになってきた．そのため講義で学んだ知識・技術を確実に理解できる新しい形の教科書として，理学療法領域の専門科目を網羅した「シンプル理学療法学シリーズ」が刊行された．

　そして，このたび，このシリーズと同じ理念のもとに理学療法士・作業療法士の共通基礎科目の教科書シリーズとして「シンプル理学療法学・作業療法学シリーズ」が刊行される運びとなった．

　編集にあたっては，「シンプル理学療法学シリーズ」と同様に以下の5点を特徴とし，これらを過不足のないように盛り込んだ．

1. 理学療法・作業療法の教育カリキュラムに準拠し，教育現場での使いやすさを追求する．
2. 障害を系統別に分類し，障害を引き起こす疾患の成り立ちを解説した上で，理学療法・作業療法の基礎的なガイドラインを提示する．このことにより，基本的な治療原則を間違えずに，的確な治療方法を適応できる思考を養えるようにする．
3. 実際の講義に即して，原則として1章が講義の1コマにおさまる内容にまとめる．さらに，演習，実習，PBL（問題解決型学習）の課題を取り込み，臨床関連のトピックスを「ヒント」としてコラム形式で解説する．また，エビデンスについても最新の情報を盛り込む．これらの講義のプラスアルファとなる内容を，教員が取捨選択できるような構成を目指し，さらに，学生の自習や発展学習にも対応し，臨床に対する興味へつながるように工夫する．
4. 網羅的な教科書とは異なり，理学療法士・作業療法士を目指す学生にとって必要かつ十分な知識・技術を厳選する．長文での解説は避け，箇条書きでの簡潔な解説と，豊富な図表・写真を駆使し，多彩な知識をシンプルに整理した理解しやすい紙面構成になるように努める．
5. 学生の理解を促すために，2色刷，キーワード等により重要なポイントがひとめでわかるようにする．また，予習・復習に活用できるように，「調べておこう」，「学習到達度自己評価問題」などの項目を設ける．

　また，いずれの理学療法士・作業療法士養成校で教育を受けても同等の臨床遂行能力が体得できるような，標準化かつ精選された「理学療法・作業療法教育ガイドライン＝理学療法・作業療法教育モデル・コアカリキュラム」となり得ることをめざした．これらの目的を達成するために，執筆者として各養成施設で教鞭をとられている実力派若手教員に参加いただいたことは大変に意味深いことであった．

　既存の教科書の概念を刷新した本シリーズが，学生の自己研鑽に活用されることを切望するとともに，理学療法士・作業療法士の養成教育のさらなる発展の契機となることを期待する．

　最後に，発刊・編集作業においてご尽力をいただいた諸兄に，心より感謝の意を表したい．

2017年1月

埼玉県立大学名誉教授　細田多穂

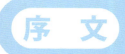

序文

　本書はリハビリテーションを専攻する英語学習者を念頭に編集された英語テキストですが，看護学など他の医療専門職を志望する学生の皆さんにも十分お使いいただける内容になっています．医療専門職を目指す学生諸君が「英語を学習する」のではなく，「英語で学習する」テキストを目指しました．全14ユニットは，理学療法学，作業療法学，英語教育学を専門とする大学教員が相談を繰り返しつつ教材化したものです．教養英語の学習段階において，既に医療専門職になるための学習が開始されていることを実感できる教材に仕上げました．

　本書の特徴として第一に挙げられる点は，医学用語の学習を重視していることです．医学用語と日本語の意味を単にリスト化するのではなく，その構造と語形成のルールをわかりやすく説明することで学習を容易にしました．たとえば，arthralgia「関節痛」という単語は，arthr-「関節」+ -algia「痛み」= arthralgia「関節痛」という構造になっており，単語を構成要素する2つのパーツはいずれもギリシャ語由来の連結形と呼ばれる要素です．

　第二の特徴として，本書の構成が挙げられます．第Ⅰ部は日常の授業の中心として用いられる部分ですが，医学用語関係の解説や練習問題が繰り返される構成になっています．その際，第Ⅱ部の解説や表を学習者が利用することで解答が容易になるように工夫されています．また，第Ⅱ部単独でも医学用語の基礎を学習する教材として利用できるように構成されており，学習者が医学用語の基礎を独学することも可能になっていますので，第Ⅱ部の練習問題を課題とするなど，授業の状況にあわせてさまざまな使い方をすることも可能です．

　全体を編集するにあたり，できるだけ平易な説明をすること，医学用語の構造を分析的に解説し，その学習を体系的に取り入れること，基本構文の定着を図ること，という3点を特に重視しました．一方，ディクテーション問題や各ユニットのトピックに関して英語でコミュニケーションを行う活動も配置し，英語を読み，書き，聴き，話す活動のバランスにも配慮してあります．

　最後に，医学用語指導に分析的なアプローチを取り入れる教材開発を評価し，本書刊行の機会を与えてくださった細田多穂埼玉県立大学名誉教授，そして編集作業を支えてくださった南江堂の諸氏に深く感謝申し上げ，ご挨拶といたします．

　2017年1月

編集者・執筆者を代表して　飯島博之

本書の構成と使い方

本書はリハビリテーション専攻の学生をはじめとする医療系学生のための英語教科書です．編集にあたり，(a) 専門的内容をわかりやすく説明すること，(b) 医学用語の学習を体系的に取り入れること，(c) 論文の読解や執筆に必要な基本構文のパターンの定着を図ること，という3点を念頭に置きました．しかし，読解や専門用語の学習にとどまらず，英語を聴き，話す活動も組み入れ，英語の4技能（リーディング，リスニング，スピーキング，ライティング）すべてを使うように各Unitにタスクを用意してあります．

第Ⅰ部では，リハビリテーション専攻の学生にとってとくに重要であると思われる疾患やけがをとりあげた全14 Unitが用意されており，次のような構成になっています．

各Unitの構成

Reading 1：トピックであるけがや病気の典型的な症例を取り上げ，患者とそれを取り巻く家族や医療関係者に焦点を当てたストーリーに基づく読解活動です．読解前活動としての語彙学習（Vocabulary Study）と読解後の内容理解を問う真偽判定問題（Reading Comprehension）から構成されています．

Reading 2：トピックであるけがや病気に関する一般的，専門的な情報と解説，および必要とされるリハビリテーションの内容に関する読解活動です．読解前活動としての語彙学習（Vocabulary Study）と読解後の英語での質問（Comprehension Questions）から構成されています．

パーツと語源で覚える医学用語：Reading 1，Reading 2の文章で用いられている医学用語をより小さな，意味を持つ単位に分解し，それらの語源と意味を解説しました．語よりも小さな意味を持つ単位（接辞，連結形）での意味を考えることで医学用語が非常に覚えやすくなります．語源をさかのぼり医学用語の意味を考える楽しさを感じていただければと思います．複数のUnitに再登場する重要語彙に関しては，参照すべきUnitを表示してありますので，関連Unitの同欄を参照し，より詳しい情報を得てください．

Dictation：本文中で用いられている構文に関連したリスニング問題です（空欄補充形式）．

Composition：本文中で用いられた構文や重要表現に関係する並べ替え英作文問題です．

Medical Terms：辞書や第Ⅱ部の語彙リスト（表1～3）を参考に，本文中で用いられた医学用語に関連のある問題に解答しながら医学用語の基礎知識を修得できるように配慮されています．

Let's Try!：取り上げた症例やけがに関して情報を交換したり，議論したりする発展的なコミュニケーション活動です．各Unitのトピックについて，覚えた用語や構文を使い，英語で話してみましょう．

第Ⅰ部で扱う文章には専門用語が多く用いられており，内容的にも専門性が伴うため，ともすれば読

解だけの活動になりがちです．まず，モデルリーディングを聴いて，Vocabulary Study の語（句）の発音練習をしっかりと行ってください．そのうえで，Reading 1, 2 については質問の答えを探す読解活動だけでなく，モデルリーディングの発音にならい，イントネーションや語句の区切りに注意しつつ，音読の練習もしてみましょう．Dictation では本文中に用いられた表現が扱われていますが，本文の英語は見ずに，モデルリーディングを聴いただけで空欄に書き込めるようにしましょう．

　第Ⅱ部は，第Ⅰ部で扱った医学用語関連の練習問題に解答するための資料として用いることができるだけでなく，医学用語に関心を持った学習者が独学できるように構成されています．第Ⅰ部で取り上げた医学用語に限定せず，医学用語全般にわたって扱っていますので，リハビリテーションに限らず，看護学等の医療分野を専攻する学生の皆さんにも十分ご活用いただけるはずです．「一目瞭然，視覚的に理解する．」という方針のもと，医学用語の理解に必要なポイントを簡潔に図解して説明しました．さらに，練習問題に解答することで知識を確認し定着できるようになっています．表1は重要な語彙パーツをアルファベット順にまとめており，辞書代わりに利用できます．表2と表3はそれぞれ，単語を分解した際に，前方にくる要素と後方にくる要素を関連する項目ごとに分類したものです．表1〜3を辞書代わりにご活用ください．

　リハビリテーションに関係したトピックを読み，聴き，書き，話す活動を通じて，英語の総合的能力を身につけることに加え，医療系学生に必要な医学用語とその関連知識も身につけていただけることを願っています．

こちらの QR コードからモデルリーディングおよび Dictation のダウンロードサイトにアクセスできます．

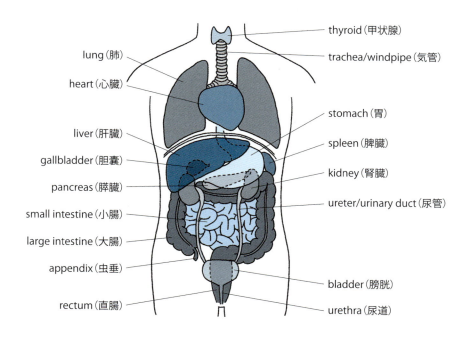
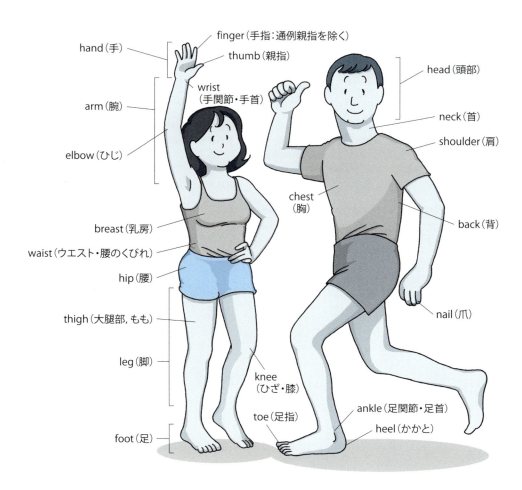

診療科と専門職

診療科名 (五十音順)	ふりがな	英語診療科名	専門職名	英語専門職名
胃腸科/ 消化器内科	いちょうか/ しょうかきないか	gastroenterology	胃腸科医	gastroenterologist
眼科	がんか	ophthalmology	眼科医	ophthalmologist
緩和医療	かんわいりょう	palliative medicine	緩和医療専門医	palliative care doctor/ palliative care specialist
形成外科	けいせいげか	plastic surgery	形成外科医	plastic surgeon
外科	げか	surgery	外科医	surgeon
血液内科	けつえきないか	hematology/haematology	血液内科医	hematologist/ haematologist
口腔外科	こうくうげか	oral surgery	口腔外科医	oral surgeon
肛門科	こうもんか	proctology	肛門科医	proctologist
呼吸器内科	こきゅうきないか	respiratory medicine/ pulmonary medicine	呼吸器内科医	pulmonologist
産婦人科	さんふじんか	obstetrics & gynecology/ obstetrics & gynaecology	産婦人科医	obstetrics & gynecology doctor/ obstetrician and gynecologist/ obstetrician (産科医)/ gynecologist/gynaecologist (婦人科医)
歯科	しか	dentistry	歯科医	dentist
耳鼻咽喉科	じびいんこうか	otorhinolaryngology/ otolaryngology/ ENT	耳鼻咽喉科医	otorhinolaryngologist/otolaryngologist/ ENT doctor
循環器内科	じゅんかんきないか	cardiology	循環器内科医	cardiologist
小児科	しょうにか	pediatrics/ paediatrics	小児科医	pediatrician/ paediatrician
神経内科	しんけいないか	neurology	神経内科医	neurologist
心療内科	しんりょうないか	psychosomatic medicine	心療内科医	psychosomatic medicine physician/ psychosomatic medicine specialist
整形外科	せいけいげか	orthopedics/ orthopaedics	整形外科医	orthopedic surgeon/orthopedist
精神科	せいしんか	psychiatry	精神科医	psychiatrist
内科	ないか	internal medicine	内科医	internist/ physician
脳神経外科	のうしんけいげか	neurosurgery	脳神経外科医	neurosurgeon
泌尿器科	ひにょうきか	urology	泌尿器科医	urologist
皮膚科	ひふか	dermatology	皮膚科医	dermatologist
美容整形外科	びようせいけいげか	cosmetic surgery	美容整形外科医	cosmetic surgeon
病理診断科	びょうりしんだんか	diagnostic pathology	病理医	pathologist
放射線科	ほうしゃせんか	radiology	放射線科医	radiologist
麻酔科	ますいか	anesthesiology/ anaesthesiology	麻酔科医	anesthesiologist/ anaesthesiologist
リハビリテーション科	りはびりてーしょんか	rehabilitation medicine	リハビリテーション専門医	physiatrist
老人科/ 老年科	ろうじんか/ ろうねんか	geriatrics	老人病専門医/ 老年医学専門医	geriatrician

保健医療関係専門職

専門職名（五十音順）	ふりがな	英語専門職名
看護師	かんごし	nurse（看護師）/registered nurse（正看護師）/assistant nurse, licensed practical nurse（准看護師）/nurse practitioner（診療看護師）/certified nurse（認定看護師）/certified nurse specialist（専門看護師）
管理栄養士	かんりえいようし	registered dietitian
義肢装具士	ぎしそうぐし	prosthetist and orthotist
救急救命士	きゅうきゅうきゅうめいし	emergency medical technician/paramedic
言語聴覚士	げんごちょうかくし	speech therapist
作業療法士	さぎょうりょうほうし	occupational therapist
歯科衛生士	しかえいせいし	dental hygienist
歯科技工士	しかぎこうし	dental laboratory technician/dental technologist
視能訓練士	しのうくんれんし	orthoptist
助産師	じょさんし	midwife
診療放射線技師	しんりょうほうしゃせんぎし	radiological technologist
認定看護管理者	にんていかんごかんりしゃ	certified nurse administrator
鍼療法士	はりりょうほうし	acupuncturist
保健師	ほけんし	public health nurse
薬剤師	やくざいし	pharmacist/chemist
理学療法士	りがくりょうほうし	physical therapist/physiotherapist
臨床検査技師	りんしょうけんさぎし	clinical laboratory technician/clinical laboratory technologist/medical laboratory technologist
臨床工学技士	りんしょうこうがくぎし	clinical engineer/medical engineer
臨床心理士	りんしょうしんりし	clinical psychologist/clinical psychotherapist

Contents

第 I 部 — 1

- **Unit 1** Femoral Neck Fracture（大腿骨頸部骨折）— 飯島博之，隈元庸夫 *3*
- **Unit 2** Osteoarthritis of the Knee（変形性膝関節症）— 飯島博之，隈元庸夫 *11*
- **Unit 3** Rheumatoid Arthritis（関節リウマチ）— 飯島博之，濱口豊太 *19*
- **Unit 4** Colles' Fracture（コレス骨折）— 飯島博之，濱口豊太 *27*
- **Unit 5** Locomotive Syndrome（ロコモティブシンドローム）— 林 幸子，隈元庸夫，飯島博之 *35*
- **Unit 6** Chronic Lower Back Pain（慢性腰痛症）— 林 幸子，隈元庸夫，飯島博之 *43*
- **Unit 7** Spinal Cord Injury（脊髄損傷）— 島崎美登里，濱口豊太，飯島博之 *51*
- **Unit 8** Adjustment Disorder and Symptomatic Depression（適応障害と症候性うつ状態）— 島崎美登里，濱口豊太，飯島博之 *59*
- **Unit 9** Parkinson's Disease（パーキンソン病）— 飯島博之，隈元庸夫 *67*
- **Unit 10** Cerebrovascular Disease（脳血管障害）— 島崎美登里，濱口豊太，飯島博之 *75*
- **Unit 11** Dementia（認知症）— 島崎美登里，濱口豊太，飯島博之 *83*
- **Unit 12** Diabetes Mellitus（糖尿病）— 島崎美登里，濱口豊太，飯島博之 *91*
- **Unit 13** COPD（慢性閉塞性肺疾患）— 林 幸子，隈元庸夫，飯島博之 *99*
- **Unit 14** Cerebral Palsy（脳性麻痺）— 林 幸子，隈元庸夫，飯島博之 *107*

第 II 部　医学用語の学習 — 飯島博之 *115*

語源とパーツによる学習方法

1. はじめに：英語における学術用語の由来 …… *117*
2. 医学用語の基礎知識 …… *117*
   - 2.1　医学用語の構造と意味 …… *117*
   - 2.2　接辞(affix)と連結形(combining form) …… *119*
   - 2.3　連結母音(combining vowel) -o- / -i- …… *121*

練習問題 …… *123*

参考文献/参照辞書/略号一覧 …… *132*

表 1 …… *134*

表 2 …… *148*

表 3 …… *159*

Index — *163*

第 I 部

Unit 1

Femoral Neck Fracture（大腿骨頸部骨折）

　大腿骨頸部骨折は大腿骨の付け根に近い部分の骨折です．骨粗鬆症が進んだ高齢者や女性に多くみられますが，今後，高齢化が進むにつれてますます増加することが予想されます．高齢者の場合，骨折により体を動かさなくなったことが原因となり，身体の筋が衰えて寝たきりになったり，認知症が進行したりするなどの合併症が発生する場合も多いので，早期の手術と早期のリハビリテーション，早期離床が重要とされています．

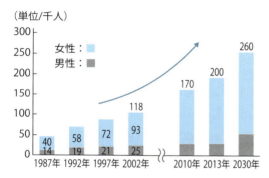

今後予測される大腿骨頸部骨折患者の数

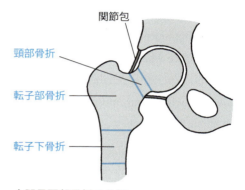

大腿骨頸部骨折の分類

Reading 1

Vocabulary Study

以下の①〜⑩の語（句）の意味を a.〜j. から選びましょう．そのうえで実際に発音を練習してみましょう．

① diagnose　　　　　a. 骨折
② fracture　　　　　 b. 大腿骨
③ femur　　　　　　c. 手術部位
④ orthopedic　　　　d. 診断する
⑤ hospitalize　　　　e. 〜を入院させる
⑥ prescribe　　　　　f.（不愉快なことを）経験する，（治療などを）受ける
⑦ dislocation　　　　g. 整形外科の
⑧ undergo　　　　　h. 大腿部
⑨ surgical site　　　 i. 処方する
⑩ femoral area　　　 j. 脱臼

Kiyomi Kaneko is a 76-year-old woman living in Sapporo, Hokkaido. She lives in a single-family house with her husband. She has two adult daughters living in Tokyo. Until recently, Mrs. Kaneko was generally healthy and was able to do household chores.

In early April this year, however, Mrs. Kaneko slipped and fell on a wet sidewalk on her way back from a nearby supermarket. She tried hard to stand up, but was unable to do so. She was taken to hospital by ambulance and was diagnosed as having a fracture of the neck of her left femur. After the diagnosis, her doctor explained to her about the extent of her injury and the need for the operation of femoral head replacement scheduled for the next day. She was also told that proper physical therapy would be essential after the operation so that she would be able to get back to normal as soon as possible.

Mako Asai is a physical therapist fresh from college and is working at the orthopedic hospital where Mrs. Kaneko was hospitalized and underwent the operation. Mako has been serving as an assistant to other senior physical therapists, and she has not had her own patient since she started working at the hospital in April. But this morning, Mako was assigned to Kiyomi Kaneko and is now determined to do her best to put into practice what she has learned for her first patient.

The postoperative rehabilitation protocol prescribed by the doctor included learning how to safely transfer to a wheelchair, muscle training of her lower limbs, and training to walk. The surgeon reminded Mako about three points that she should remember regarding Kaneko's medical rehabilitation. First, Mako needed to be careful to avoid dislocation of the hip prosthesis as Mrs. Kaneko had undergone femoral head replacement. The second point was that the weight load in the exercise program could be progressively increased until the patient felt pain. The third point was the importance of preventing her from falling by providing her with balance training.

Mako visited Mrs. Kaneko in bed after her operation and explained that she was in charge of her rehabilitation program scheduled to start the next day. At that time, Mrs. Kaneko was icing the surgical site of her femoral area. She was also learning from an experienced nurse how to prevent a dislocation when rolling over and how to sit up in bed. Mako explained that Mrs. Kaneko's medical rehabilitation protocol was going to start by doing exactly what she had just learned from the nurse. After talking with Mrs. Kaneko and the nurse, Mako decided to start Mrs. Kaneko's physical therapy in her hospital room at 10 a.m. the next day.

Notes: **single-family house** 一戸建て住宅, **hip prosthesis** 人工股関節, **femoral head replacement** 人工骨頭置換術, **protocol** プロトコル, （患者の治療を実行するための）計画.

Reading Comprehension

本文の内容に一致するものにはT（True），異なるものにはF（False）を記入しましょう．

① Kiyomi lives with her husband and daughters in Sapporo.　（　　）
② Kiyomi was able to stand up with difficulty when she fell down on the wet sidewalk.　（　　）
③ Kiyomi fell down and fractured the neck of her right femur.　（　　）
④ Kiyomi's doctor decided to replace her left hip joint with an artificial joint.　（　　）
⑤ The doctor asked Mako to gradually increase the weight load during Kiyomi's rehabilitation even if Kiyomi felt pain.　（　　）
⑥ Kiyomi first learned from Mako about how to prevent a dislocation of the hip prosthesis.　（　　）
⑦ Mako is an experienced physical therapist who can deal with any condition.　（　　）
⑧ A patient who has undergone femoral head replacement needs to be careful of dislocation of the hip prosthesis.　（　　）
⑨ Mako asked a nurse to teach Kiyomi how to sit up in bed.　（　　）
⑩ Mako is going to start Kiyomi's rehabilitation by teaching her how to roll over properly and sit up in bed.　（　　）

パーツと語源で覚える医学用語

● **orthopedic（orthopaedic）整形外科の**

　フランス語 *orthopédie* に由来．orth(o)- は「まっすぐな（straight），正しい（right, correct）」の意でギリシャ語 *orthos*（straight, right）が語源．*orthos*（straight, right）＋ *paideia*（rearing of children）という構造となり，本来は「子供の体の変形を予防，矯正するための術」を意味したと考えられています．

● **postoperative 手術後の**

　post- は「（時間的・空間的に）後の」の意．ラテン語 *post*（after, behind）に由来．operative は「手術の」の意の形容詞．
＊preoperative の意味を推測してから第Ⅱ部の表や辞書で意味を確認してみましょう．

Reading 2

Vocabulary Study

以下の①～⑩の語（句）の意味を a. ～ j. から選びましょう．そのうえで実際に発音を練習してみましょう．

① arthralgia　　　　　　　a. 可動性
② mobility　　　　　　　　b. 筋の
③ bedridden　　　　　　　c. 歩行
④ dementia　　　　　　　 d. 下肢
⑤ postoperative　　　　　 e. 手術後の
⑥ ambulation　　　　　　 f. 可動域
⑦ muscular　　　　　　　 g. 関節痛
⑧ lower limb　　　　　　　h. 寝たきりの
⑨ deterioration　　　　　　i. 認知症
⑩ range of motion　　　　 j. 低下，悪化

　　A femoral neck fracture is a condition characterized by a break in the neck of the femur or thighbone. It is a common condition in the elderly, who have a higher risk of falling and fracture because they are more likely to have poor balance. One of the characteristic complaints associated with this injury is intense pain at the site of the fracture. In the case of an elderly person, arthralgia, or joint pain, tends to restrict the patient's mobility, which can cause the patient to end up being bedridden. In the worst case, bedridden elderly people might develop dementia as a result of being confined to bed all day.

　　Early postoperative ambulation is the key to the prevention of these undesirable consequences. In order to prevent elderly people from being bedridden and developing dementia, early postoperative rehabilitation, including training in sitting and standing positions, is important. However, bone fusion requires time, especially in the case of a femoral neck fracture in an elderly person.

　　Therefore, operative treatments like femoral head replacement（FHR）are a likely choice（Figure 1）. Dislocation of the hip prosthesis is of great concern during postoperative recovery. This condition is most likely to occur when a patient rolls over after an operation for FHR. Therefore, the patient is sometimes advised to place a pillow between his legs if his understanding of the risk of the movement is inadequate or he has pronounced muscular weakness（Figure 2）.

　　Straight-leg-raising exercises are common in postoperative rehabilitation（Figure 3）. Exercises such as plantar flexion and dorsiflexion aimed at improving the blood circulation of the injured lower limb and the perception of sensation in the plantar surface are also common. Training of the hip abductor muscles is also needed to increase the stability of the injured lower limb.

　　Patients who suffer femoral neck fractures and undergo surgery often have difficulty in carrying out the activities of daily living. They need to make up for the deterioration in the function of their lower limbs by using other parts of the body. As the elderly tend to lack enough muscle strength, they should be trained systematically in postoperative rehabilitation programs. For example, patients need to strengthen the abdominal muscles needed for the act of sitting up. They also need enough joint range of motion of both lower limbs and muscle strength for transfer motion. To use parallel bars and crutches, patients need enough muscle strength in their upper limbs. Postoperative training in walking usually starts with partial weight bearing, and gradually advances to full weight bearing. Due to improved surgical techniques, however, it is not uncommon today to start walking exercises with full weight bearing the next day after surgery.

Notes：**plantar flexion** 底屈，**dorsiflexion** 背屈，**the perception of sensation in the plantar surface** 足底の感覚（知覚），**hip abductor muscles** 股関節外転筋，**activities of daily living** 日常生活活動（ADL），**abdominal muscles** 腹筋，**transfer motion** 移乗動作，**partial weight bearing** 部分荷重，**full weight bearing** 全荷重．

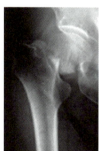
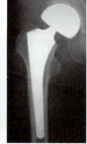
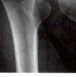

大腿骨頸部骨折　　人工骨頭置換術
Figure 1． 大腿骨のX線画像

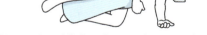
Figure 2． 手術後の寝返り（roll over）の方法

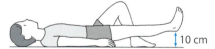
Figure 3． 手術後のトレーニング方法

Comprehension Questions

以下の問いに英語で答えましょう．

① What is a femoral neck fracture?
② Who is more likely to suffer the condition? And why?
③ What can happen to the elderly in the worst case as a result of being confined to bed all day?
④ What is the key to avoiding becoming bedridden and developing dementia?
⑤ What should early postoperative rehabilitation include?
⑥ Why is femoral head replacement a likely choice in treating an elderly person?
⑦ What should patients be careful of during recovery from the operation of femoral head replacement?
⑧ What are exercises such as plantar flexion and dorsiflexion for?
⑨ In the activities of daily living, how do patients make up for the deterioration in the function of their lower limbs?
⑩ How does ambulation exercise usually start?

パーツと語源で覚える医学用語

● **arthralgia** 関節痛
arthr(o)- は「関節（joint）」の意の連結形．ギリシャ語 *arthron*（joint）が語源．-algia は「痛み（pain）」の意のギリシャ語 *algos* 由来の後部連結形．母音 a で始まっているので前部連結形は arthr- となり，連結母音 -o- は現れない．

● **dementia** 認知症
ラテン語 *dementem*（out of one's mind）「正気を失って」が語源．-ia は名詞を作る接尾辞．病名にも多い．

● **muscular** 筋の
muscul(o)- は「筋」の意の連結形．ラテン語 *musculus*（muscle）が語源．-ar は形容詞を作るラテン語系接尾辞．
*the musculoskeletal system の和訳はどうなるか考えてみましょう．

● **dorsiflexion** 背屈
dorsi- は「背面の」の意の連結形．ラテン語 *dorsum*（back）に由来．flexion は手足・関節の屈曲（運動）．dors(o)- も同じ意味．cf. dorsolateral（背面側部の）

Dictation

録音を聴いて空欄を埋め，各英文を完成させましょう．

① A (　　　　　　　　　　　　　　　　　　　　　　　) in the elderly.

② Early (　　　　　　　　　　　　　　　　) of these undesirable consequences.

③ Patients need enough (　　　　　　　　　　　　　　　　　) to use the device.

Composition

日本語の意味に合うように〔　〕内の語（句）を並べ替えましょう．必要に応じて「,」を使用してください．

① 高橋さんは人間ドックに入った際に前立腺癌だと診断された．

Mr. Takahashi〔 diagnosed, was, having, as, prostate cancer, when, he, hospitalized, was 〕for a physical checkup.

② この病院は来年中には完成の予定である．

This〔 is, scheduled, hospital, the next year, completed, be, to, within 〕.

③ 喫煙の習慣がある人のほうがはるかに肺がんにかかりやすい．

Habitual〔 likely, far more, to, lung, smokers, are, develop 〕cancer.

④ 私がメアリーを訪ねたとき，彼女の父は関節炎で寝たきりだった．

When I visited Mary,〔 father, bedridden, her, was, arthritis, with 〕.

⑤ HIV にかかった人が，診断の直後に落ち込んでしまうことは珍しくはない．

It is〔 with HIV, not, people, to, depressed, uncommon, for, feel 〕soon after the diagnosis is made.

⑥ 肝炎とは肝臓の炎症を特徴とする疾患である．

Hepatitis〔 characterized, inflammation, a disease, is, by, the liver, of 〕.

⑦ 塩分控えめが健康の鍵だ．

Moderate〔 of, health, key, consumption, salt, good, is, the, to 〕.

⑧ 医者は彼に脂っこい食品を食べないようにと助言した．

The〔 advised, doctor, him, foods, not, fatty, to, eat 〕.

⑨ 栄養の偏った食事と運動不足の結果，生活習慣病になる人がますます増えている．

More and more〔 lifestyle-related, developing, poor, a result, people, are, diseases, as, of, diet 〕and lack of exercise.

⑩ 医学の進歩のおかげで発達障害のある人がより長く生きられるようになってきている．

Owing〔 to, medical, individuals, with, longer, advances, disabilities, are now, living, developmental 〕.

Medical Terms

第Ⅱ部のリスト（表1～3）を参考に，以下のフローチャートの空欄を埋めましょう．

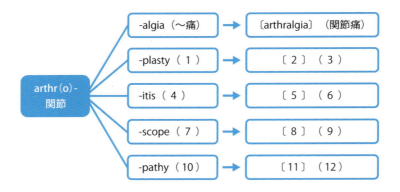

Let's try!

Suppose you live with an 80-year-old grandmother, what would you do to minimize her risk of suffering a fractured femoral neck? Talk with your partner in English.

パーツと語源で覚える医学用語

● 連結形（combining form）と連結母音（combining vowel）の基礎知識

　上のフローチャートでは「関節」を意味する要素 arthr(o)- で始まる医学用語を調べました．この arthr(o)- は連結形（combining form）と呼ばれ，ギリシャ語に由来する意味を持つ要素で，独立語としては存在せず，他の語，連結形，接辞と結び付くことで成立する形式です．

　arthr(o)- において（　）で表示されている母音 -o- は連結母音と呼ばれます．連結母音は前後2つの要素をつなげる役割を果たしますが，原則として，後続の要素が子音で始まっている場合に現れ，母音で始まっている場合には現れません．連結母音 -o- は本来，ギリシャ語系の要素を結合する際に用いられた母音です．ラテン語での連結母音は -i- が用いられていましたが，ギリシャ語系語彙がラテン語へ取り入れられ同化するに伴い，ギリシャ語で用いられていた -o- がラテン語の要素間，あるいは，ギリシャ語とラテン語の要素間の連結においても用いられるようになり，今日では連結母音 -o- が広く用いられています．なお，連結母音 -o- は通常，前部連結形に付加されているものとして扱われ，医学用語集などでは arthr(o)- や arthr/o- のように提示されています．また，多くの辞書では arthro-，arthr- のようにそれぞれを見出しとして表示しています．連結形と連結母音について，詳しくは第Ⅱ部をご覧ください．

Unit 2

Osteoarthritis of the Knee（変形性膝関節症）

　変形性膝関節症には，加齢に伴う一次性のものと外傷や炎症などにより生じる二次性のものがありますが，年齢とともに多くなり，女性や肥満の人に比較的多くみられる病気です．初期症状としては，膝のこわばり，歩き始め，階段の昇降や長時間の歩行後の痛みなどがあり，炎症が強い場合は，初期であっても強い痛みを伴う場合があります．膝の変形が進行するにつれて，正座や膝の屈伸が困難になり，痛みや歩行障害のために日常生活が制限されるようになります．O脚（bowlegged）やX脚（knock-kneed）といった変形が生じるケースもみられます．

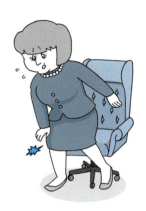

立ち上がりや歩きはじめに膝が痛む（休めば痛みはとれる）．

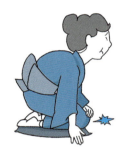

歩くと膝が痛み，正座や階段の昇り降りが困難．

Reading 1

Vocabulary Study

以下の①～⑩の語（句）の意味をa.～j.から選びましょう．そのうえで実際に発音を練習してみましょう．

① enthusiastic		a.	（病気・症状の）悪化
② inevitable		b.	避けられない，不可避の
③ bowlegged		c.	熱心な
④ therapy		d.	変形性関節症（骨関節炎）
⑤ dormitory		e.	寄宿舎，寮
⑥ walkable		f.	軽減する，緩和する
⑦ exacerbation		g.	O脚の
⑧ orthopedist		h.	歩いて行ける
⑨ osteoarthritis		i.	治療，療法
⑩ alleviate		j.	整形外科医

Unit 2　Osteoarthritis of the Knee（変形性膝関節症）

　　Takako Ishii is a 71-year-old woman living in Saitama City, Saitama Prefecture. She lives in her own house with her husband. She used to enjoy physical activities and played sports when she was younger. She had been an enthusiastic member of a community volleyball team until the age of 50. However, she gradually gained weight after she stopped playing volleyball and weighs over 75 kilograms now. She is aware that her leg muscles are much weaker and easily gets tired after walking up and down the stairs. There were times when she felt pain in her knee joints, but she accepted such symptoms as an inevitable change caused by aging. But she started to feel pain in her knees more frequently, and one day she noticed that she was bowlegged. These changes made her take her conditions more seriously.

　　Miho Tanaka, a granddaughter of Takako, is a sophomore majoring in physical therapy in university. Miho lives alone in the dormitory of her university, which is within a walkable distance from Takako's house. One day, Miho went shopping with her grandmother and noticed that Takako's pace of walking was much slower than usual. When Miho asked Takako about her unusual slow pace of walking, she complained of the pain in her knees when walking over a long distance or walking up and down the stairs. As Miho had already learned the basics of rehabilitation as a physical therapy major, she felt that she should do something to relieve Takako's leg pain and prevent future exacerbation.

　　The next day, Miho visited Prof. Suzuki, one of the physical therapy professors at her university, to ask for some advice. She explained to him about her grandmother's condition and asked him what she should do for her grandmother. After asking Miho a few questions about Takako's symptoms, Prof. Suzuki advised Miho to take her grandmother to an orthopedist at her earliest convenience as it was highly likely that her grandmother was suffering from osteoarthritis of the knee judging from Miho's story. He also advised Miho to tell her grandmother to lose weight and build muscular strength to improve the conditions. The professor also added that icing would alleviate her arthralgia to some extent.

　　Miho visited her grandmother on her way back to the dormitory and conveyed to her Prof. Suzuki's advice. Miho also told Takako that she was going to accompany Takako to an orthopedic hospital when it was convenient for the both of them. Takako appreciated her granddaughter's kindness and thought that she was very lucky to have a granddaughter studying rehabilitation.

Notes：at one's earliest convenience　できるだけ早く，都合がつき次第.

Reading Comprehension

本文の内容に一致するものには T（True），異なるものには F（False）を記入しましょう．

① Takako loved sports when she was younger.　（　　）
② Takako started playing volleyball at the age of 50.　（　　）
③ Takako started to gain weight because playing volleyball increased her appetite.　（　　）
④ Takako realizes that she has lost the muscular strength of her legs.　（　　）
⑤ At first, Takako thought that her knee joint pain was an unavoidable condition that elderly people have to bear.　（　　）
⑥ One day, Takako realized a change in the shape of her legs.　（　　）
⑦ Takako's granddaughter majors in rehabilitation in university.　（　　）
⑧ Miho's professor suggested that Takako should see an orthopedist as soon as possible.　（　　）
⑨ Prof. Suzuki said that Takako's joint pain would be relieved to some degree by icing.　（　　）
⑩ Miho decided to take her grandmother to an orthopedic hospital whether she wanted to go or not.　（　　）

パーツと語源で覚える医学用語

● **osteoarthritis**　変形性関節症（骨関節炎）

　oste(o)- は「骨（bone）」の意のギリシャ語 *osteon* に由来する連結形．arthr(o)- は「関節（joint）」の意のギリシャ語由来の前部連結形，-itis は「～炎（inflammatory disease）」の意のギリシャ語由来の接尾辞．よって，oste(o)-＋arthr(o)-＋-itis の構造から文字どおり和訳すると「骨関節炎」となります．英語名には「変形性」にあたる要素が含まれていませんが，今日の臨床においては変形性関節症の呼び方が広く使われています．なお，osteoarthritis のスペリングですが，後続の arthritis が母音で始まっているにもかかわらず，osteo- 部分の連結母音 -o- が現れ，ostearthritis とはなっていません．語末要素である接尾辞 -itis と連結する arthr(o)- のみ連結母音 -o- が不要になります．詳しくは，第Ⅱ部の図5と解説を参照してください．

Reading 2

Vocabulary Study

以下の①～⑩の語（句）の意味を a.～j. から選びましょう．そのうえで実際に発音を練習してみましょう．

① degenerative　　　　a. こわばり
② cartilage　　　　　　b.（病気などの）発病，発症
③ stiffness　　　　　　c. 治療（上）の
④ stage　　　　　　　　d. 持続性の
⑤ onset　　　　　　　　e. 保存的な
⑥ deformity　　　　　　f. 段階
⑦ genetics　　　　　　g. 変形，奇形
⑧ persistent　　　　　h. 変性の，退行性の
⑨ conservative　　　　i. 遺伝（現象）
⑩ therapeutic　　　　　j. 軟骨

　Osteoarthritis of the knee is a degenerative disease of the knee joints in which cartilage, the natural cushioning between joints, wears out over time, resulting in the development of osteophytes and cysts at the margins of the knee joints. The main symptoms of the disorder may include joint pain, swelling, feeling of warmth in the joint, stiffness in the joint, decrease in joint mobility, and a grating sensation heard or felt when the knees are moved.

　During the early stage of the disease, there is pain in the knee joints when standing up or walking, but the pain disappears on resting for a while. If such symptoms are overlooked at the onset of the disease, the disorder can advance to the middle stage, in which joint pain is felt more frequently, and there is difficulty sitting straight with legs folded under you and walking up and down the stairs. In the advanced stage, the meniscus, a primary shock absorber in the knee, wears away severely, which can result in noticeable knee deformity. The Japanese are thought to be more likely to develop bowlegs than knock knees. In this stage, the knees cannot be straightened and there is great difficulty carrying out activities of daily living.

　There are two types of osteoarthritis of the knee. Primary osteoarthritis, which is caused by multiple factors, is more commonly diagnosed and is considered to be related to such factors as aging, obesity, muscular weakness, etc., while secondary osteoarthritis has a specific cause such as an injury, genetics or diseases.

　Options for the treatment of osteoarthritis of the knee can be surgical or non-surgical. In the advanced stage of osteoarthritis, where knee deformity is extremely noticeable, total knee arthroplasty will be performed. This procedure can be very effective in eliminating persistent arthralgia. However, in the treatment guidelines for osteoarthritis of the knee, this procedure is usually applicable to cases in which constant arthralgia is experienced, and there is difficulty conducting activities of daily living. Therefore, conservative, or non-surgical treatment is usually the option for most cases of osteoarthritis of the knee, where therapeutic exercise and education play vital roles. There is evidence that therapeutic exercise, which can promote muscular strength, flexibility and aerobic capacity, is the most effective. Exercises usually include stretching to strengthen quadriceps and hamstring muscles, since muscles surrounding the knee joint function as shock absorbers for the pressure on the knee joint brought about by daily activities and playing sports. Aerobic exercise for weight loss can also be prescribed in an effort to decrease pressure placed on the knee joint. The use of a walking stick, lateral wedge insoles, knee supporters and knee braces would also be possible prescriptions aimed at reducing pressure on knee joints and supporting the knees.

> **Notes**：**degenerative disease** 変性疾患，**osteophyte** 骨棘（骨の異常な突起），**cyst** 嚢胞，**wear out** 擦り減る，**grating sensation** きしむような感じ，**meniscus** 半月板，**knock knees** X脚，**total knee arthroplasty（TKA）** 人工膝関節全置換術，**quadriceps** 四頭筋，**hamstring muscles** ハムストリングス，**aerobic exercise** 有酸素運動，**therapeutic exercise** 運動療法，**lateral wedge insoles** 外側楔状足底板，**knee braces** 膝装具．

Comprehension Questions

以下の問いに英語で答えましょう．

① What is osteoarthritis of the knee?
② What are the main symptoms of osteoarthritis of the knee?
③ Describe the pain patients feel at the beginning stage of osteoarthritis of the knee.
④ In the middle stage of the disease, what problems will patients have?
⑤ What is a meniscus?
⑥ In the advanced stage of osteoarthritis of the knee, what can happen to patients?
⑦ What are the risk factors for primary osteoarthritis?
⑧ In what cases is surgical treatment considered?
⑨ Why do therapeutic exercises focus on quadriceps and hamstring muscles?
⑩ Why is losing weight important for patients with osteoarthritis of the knee?

パーツと語源で覚える医学用語

● **osteophyte** 骨棘(こつきょく)，骨増殖体
　osteophyte は小さな骨の異常な隆起・突起を意味する．-phyte「病的増殖」はギリシャ語 *phuton*（plant）が語源．

● **arthroplasty** 関節形成（術）
　-plasty は「成形（formation）」「形成手術（plastic surgery）」の意．arthr(o)-「関節」に結び付いて関節形成（術）．

● **quadriceps** 四頭筋
　quadri-「4」はラテン語 *quattuor*（four）が語源．-ceps「頭が〜の，〜頭の（-headed）」と結び付いて four-headed の意．

● **prescribe** 処方する
　ラテン語 *praescribere* が語源．*prae*-「前に（pre-）」+ *scribere*「書く（write）」．

Dictation

録音を聴いて空欄を埋め，各英文を完成させましょう．

① There were times when she felt pain in her knee joints, but （　　　　　　　　　　　　　　　　） caused by aging.

② Miho noticed that Takako's （　　　　　　　　　　　　　　　　　　　　　　）.

③ The professor also added that （　　　　　　　　　　　　　　　　　　　　　　）.

Composition

日本語の意味に合うように〔　〕内の語（句）を並べ替えましょう．必要に応じて「，」を使用してください．

① その患者は胸部の鋭い痛みを訴えた．

The patient 〔 of, a, complained, pain, sharp, in 〕 his chest.

② 彼女の病状は急激に悪化し，入退院を繰り返すようになった．

Her 〔 rapidly deteriorated, in, frequent, resulting, condition, hospitalization 〕.

③ 日常生活活動はリハビリテーションにおいてセルフケアにかかわる包括的な用語として用いられる．

In rehabilitation, activities of daily living (ADL) 〔 an, as, used, umbrella term, is, relating, to 〕 self-care.

④ アメリカのがん死亡の6割以上が喫煙と食事によるものである．

More than 〔 cancer deaths, are, caused, and, diet, 60 percent, of, U.S., by, smoking 〕.

⑤ この薬は糖尿病の治療に有効な役割を果たした．

This 〔 the, diabetes, drug, played, a positive, treatment, of, role, in 〕.

⑥ 砂糖入り飲料の消費を減らすことが肥満の罹患率を減らすことになるという十分な根拠がある．

There is 〔 sugar-sweetened, beverage, reduce, the, prevalence, sufficient, evidence, that, decreasing, consumption, will 〕 of obesity.

⑦ このプログラムは生活習慣病を防ぐことが目的である．

This program 〔 becoming, diseases, is, aimed, at, preventing, victims of, lifestyle-related, people, from 〕.

⑧ その研究によると，コーヒーをたくさん飲む人は口腔がんと咽頭がんにかかりにくいことがわかった．

The study reported that 〔 a lot of, to, were, who, less, people, coffee, likely, drank, develop, cancers 〕 of the mouth and throat.

⑨ その病気の初期症状は疲労，微熱，そして食欲不振である．

The initial 〔 of, the disease, include, fatigue, mild fever, and loss, symptoms, of, appetite 〕.

⑩ うつ病の原因は不明であるが，多くの要因がその発症に関係していると考えられている．

The exact cause of depression is not known, but 〔 considered, to, development, number, of, factors, be, related, to, its, a, are 〕.

Medical Terms

（A）第Ⅱ部のリスト（表1〜3）を参考に，以下のフローチャートの空欄を埋めましょう．

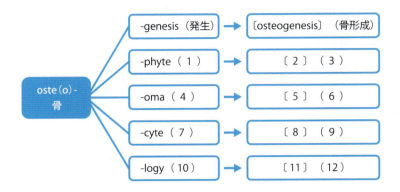

（B）下の各パーツの意味を調べてから，〔1〕〜〔6〕に適するパーツや語を入れましょう．

oste(o)-　　（意味：　　　　　　　　）
sarc(o)-　　（意味：　　　　　　　　）
chondr(o)-　（意味：　　　　　　　　）
-oma　　　　（意味：　　　　　　　　）

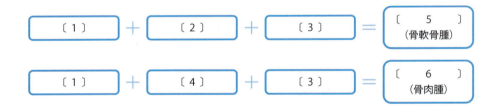

Let's try!

　Make pairs and perform a short skit. One person will play the role of a stubborn grandfather who refuses to go to an orthopedic hospital in spite of his knee joint pain. The other person will play the role of his child who tries to persuade him to go to a hospital.

Unit 3

Rheumatoid Arthritis（関節リウマチ）

　関節リウマチは誰にでも発生しますが，とくに女性に多くの患者がみられます．関節の炎症により，こわばり，痛み，腫れが生じ，進行すると関節の変形や機能障害につながる病気です．関節の炎症が長期にわたると関節が破壊され変形や強直（きょうちょく）を生じ，日常生活活動が著しく制限されることになるため，早期の診断と適切な治療が重要です．

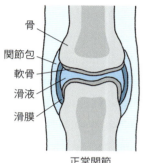
正常関節

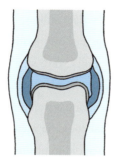
関節包と軟骨に病変が生じた関節

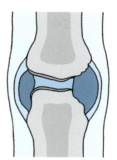
炎症増殖した滑膜と骨変形した関節

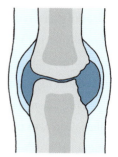
軟骨が消失して骨破壊が進んだ関節

関節リウマチにみられる関節変形の機序

Reading 1

Vocabulary Study

以下の①〜⑩の語（句）の意味を a.〜j. から選びましょう．そのうえで実際に発音を練習してみましょう．

① homemaker　　　　　　a. 炎症性の，炎症を伴う
② attending physician　　b. 関節の
③ chronic　　　　　　　　c. 補助器具
④ waterproof　　　　　　 d. 防水の
⑤ ready-made　　　　　　e. 主婦
⑥ assistive device　　　　f. 日常の仕事
⑦ articular　　　　　　　　g. 主治医（担当医）
⑧ inflammatory　　　　　 h. 既製品の
⑨ daily chores　　　　　　i. 慢性の
⑩ acknowledge　　　　　　j. 承認する

Unit 3 Rheumatoid Arthritis（関節リウマチ）

Junko Tanaka is a 50-year-old homemaker living in a suburban single-family house with her husband and three children. She first noticed a change in her wrist joints in the morning about a year ago. She started to feel stiffness in her wrists after getting out of bed, and the stiffness gradually increased, slowing down her morning routine. She also felt warmth in her wrist joints when cooking. She did not take these changes too seriously at first, but then joint pain developed. The joint pain gradually increased in severity until it became unbearable. This made her take her condition more seriously and she decided to go to an orthopedist. She conducted a Web search on the painful stiffness of her wrist joints and came to suspect she had arthropathy before going to the hospital. At the hospital, she was diagnosed as having rheumatoid arthritis（RA）as she had expected, but emotionally she had been prepared to accept the reality.

Hiroshi Mizuno is an occupational therapist working for the hospital where Junko was diagnosed as having RA. Hiroshi received instructions from Junko's attending physician and was put in charge of her. Hiroshi measured the ranges of motion of her fingers, wrists, elbows, and shoulders with a goniometer after asking her some questions about her daily life to gather information about her condition. Junko had difficulty cooking and cleaning especially when her joints were stiff and painful in the morning. She hoped that the chronic pain she felt in the activities of daily living would be relieved as soon as possible.

Hiroshi suggested that Junko do her daily chores wearing a waterproof wrist band to protect her hand joints. This was a simple ready-made assistive device that could be used for her kitchen work. Hiroshi also taught her how to use her hands in her daily activities to avoid imposing needless mechanical stress on the joints of her fingers and hands, as mechanical stress can result in the damage of the articular cartilage tissue when blood tests show the inflammatory reaction of RA. Junko needed to live with the disorder with a minimum amount of articular motion until her symptoms could be eased. Hiroshi suggested that Junko reduce the burden of housework to provide herself with enough rest. Junko listened to his advice and explanation about how to live with the disorder. She told him that she would ask her husband and children to help her with her daily chores, but she wished to at least prepare meals for her family, as doing housework, especially cooking, was a labor of love. Hiroshi listened to her and acknowledged her wishes. This is why Junko started to practice how to hold pans and knives with both hands.

Notes：**arthropathy** 関節症，関節疾患，**goniometer** 角度計（ゴニオメーター），**articular motion** 関節運動，**labor of love** 好きでする仕事．

Reading Comprehension

本文の内容に一致するものにはT（True），異なるものにはF（False）を記入しましょう．

① Junko Tanaka lives in an apartment with her husband and three children.　（　　）
② The stiffness Junko Tanaka felt in her wrist joints gradually increased and affected her activities of daily living.　（　　）
③ Junko's joint pain was extremely intense even when she started to feel warmth in her wrist joints.　（　　）
④ Junko collected information about the condition of her wrist joints before going to an orthopedist.　（　　）
⑤ Junko's condition was diagnosed as rheumatoid arthritis.　（　　）
⑥ Hiroshi is the orthopedist who is in charge of Junko.　（　　）
⑦ Hiroshi examined to what extent Junko could move her joints of fingers, wrists, elbows, and shoulders.　（　　）
⑧ Hiroshi gave Junko some advice to make her daily life easier.　（　　）
⑨ Junko needed to consider how to live with rheumatoid arthritis.　（　　）
⑩ Junko did not enjoy doing housework but Hiroshi advised her to do some daily chores so that she could have some regularity in her daily life.　（　　）

パーツと語源で覚える医学用語

● **orthopedist/orthopaedist**　整形外科医（Unit 1を参照）
　-ist は「〜をする人，専門家，〜主義者」の意の接尾辞．orth(o)- は「まっすぐな，正しい」の意．

● **diagnose**　診断する
　diagnosis「診断」からの逆成語．接頭辞 dia-「離れて」+ -gnosis「認識」= diagnosis「診断」．-gnosis は「知識（knowledge）・認識（recognition）」の意の後部連結形．ギリシャ語 *gnosis*（knowledge）に由来．cf. prognosis「予後」

● **arthropathy**　関節症，関節疾患
　-pathy は「病気（disease）」や「療法（treatment）」の意のギリシャ語由来の後部連結形．arthr(o)-「関節（joint）」に結び付いて関節疾患の意．arthr(o)- は Unit 1 を参照．

● **rheumatoid**　リウマチ性
　rheumat(o)- は「リウマチ」の意の連結形．ギリシャ語 *rheuma*（flow）に由来．-oid は「〜のようなもの，〜状のもの，〜質のもの」の意の接尾辞．ギリシャ語 *eidos*（form）に由来．古代ギリシャでは脳から流れ出す悪い液体が関節にたまり痛みが生じると考えた．

● **arthritis**　関節炎
　-itis は「〜炎（inflammation）」の意のギリシャ語由来の接尾辞．

● **goniometer**　角度計（ゴニオメーター）
　goni(o)-「角・隅」はギリシャ語 *gonia*（angle）に由来する前部連結形．-meter は「〜計，計器」．

Reading 2

Vocabulary Study

以下の①〜⑩の語（句）の意味を a.〜j. から選びましょう．そのうえで実際に発音を練習してみましょう．

① affect　　　　　　　　a. 包括的な
② symmetrical　　　　　b. 抑制する
③ immune　　　　　　　c. 医薬品，薬物
④ comprehensive　　　　d. （病気などが）〜を冒す，襲う
⑤ control　　　　　　　 e. 対称性の
⑥ potent　　　　　　　 f. 効力のある，よく効く
⑦ medication　　　　　 g. 〜に対処する
⑧ dose　　　　　　　　 h. 副作用
⑨ side effect　　　　　　i. 免疫
⑩ address　　　　　　　j. 服用量，投与量

　Rheumatoid arthritis (RA) is an autoimmune disorder that commonly affects the joints of the hands, wrists, elbows, knees, feet and ankles. The effect of the disease is usually symmetrical, which means that if one hand is affected, the other one is also affected. RA occurs when the immune system mistakenly attacks healthy body tissues. It is a chronic inflammatory disease that typically causes a painful swelling in the joints and can result in articular deformities and dysfunction in the advanced stage. RA affects about one percent of the world population. It can happen to people of all ages but most commonly begins between ages 30 and 50, and women are nearly three times more likely to get RA than men are.

　As RA is a chronic disease for which there is no cure, the treatment is now aimed at achieving remission, minimizing joint damage, and improving physical function and quality of life. Therefore, a comprehensive program consisting of medical, social and emotional support for the patient is required for the optimal treatment of RA. Some drugs are used to control the production of inflammatory substances and slow or stop the progress of the disease, but nonsteroidal anti-inflammatory drugs (NSAIDs) are usually selected as the first choice to ease arthritis pain and inflammation. Corticosteroids are also known to be potent and quick-acting anti-inflammatory medications, but doctors prefer to use them only when necessary, at the lowest dose possible and for the shortest duration of time because of the risk of side effects. They can even adversely affect patients' vital prognoses if used for prolonged periods.

　Surgery for RA can be an important option for patients with severe damage that restricts their mobility and independence. Replacement arthroplasty, which involves replacing damaged parts of a joint with metal and plastic parts, can relieve pain and restore function of joints severely damaged by RA.

　Rehabilitation plays a significant part in the management of the disease. Patients with RA need to learn about their physical symptoms and how to address those symptoms using assistive devices such as mobility aids and hand splints. Physical and occupational therapists teach RA patients how to conduct activities of daily living to avoid joint damage and destruction. For example, RA patients may be advised to sling their bags over their arms or hold them with both hands to minimize pressure on finger joints. Physical therapists can help to design proper exercise programs considering patients' needs and conditions. On the other hand, occupational therapists are more focused on helping patients with practical strategies for achieving everyday tasks. Occupational therapists can provide significant benefits for patients with RA by helping them overcome their physical limitations so that they can live independently and maintain a good quality of life.

> **Notes**：**remission** 寛解（疾患の症状が緩和・消失している状態），**optimal treatment** 最適治療，**corticosteroids** コルチコステロイド，**vital prognoses** 生命予後（単数形は prognosis），**replacement arthroplasty** 関節置換術，**mobility aids** 移動補助具，**hand splints** 手装具．

Comprehension Questions

以下の問いに英語で答えましょう．
① When does RA occur?
② What are typical symptoms of RA?
③ What percentage of the world population suffers from RA?
④ Who are more likely to be affected by RA?
⑤ What is the goal of the treatment for RA?
⑥ What should a comprehensive treatment program for RA include?
⑦ What drugs are commonly prescribed for RA as the first choice?
⑧ Why do doctors prefer to use corticosteroids for the shortest duration of time in spite of their remarkable effect on RA?
⑨ What is replacement arthroplasty?
⑩ What do RA patients need to learn about in rehabilitation?

パーツと語源で覚える医学用語

- **autoimmune** 自己免疫（性）の
  aut(o)- は「自己の（self）」の意のギリシャ語 *autos* に由来．auto- ＋immune「免疫（性）の」で「自己免疫（性）の」の意の形容詞．

- **dysfunction** 機能障害
  dys- は「悪化・不良（bad），困難（difficult）」の意のギリシャ語由来の前部連結形．dys- ＋ function「機能」＝「機能障害」．

- **nonsteroidal** 非ステロイド性の
  non- は「非，不，無（not）」の意の接頭辞．ラテン語 *non*「～でない（not）」に由来．消極的な否定や欠如を表す．

- **anti-inflammatory** 抗炎症（性）の
  anti- は「反，抗（against）」の意のラテン語由来の接頭辞．anti- ＋ inflammatory「炎症性の」＝「抗炎症（性）の」．

- **corticosteroid** コルチコステロイド（副腎皮質でつくられるステロイドの総称）
  cortic(o)- は「皮質（cortex）」の意のラテン語由来の前部連結形．とくに，大脳と副腎に関して用いられる．

- **prognosis** 予後（病気の経過・回復に関する見通し）
  -gnosis は「知識（knowledge）・認識（recognition）」の意の後部連結形．ギリシャ語 *gnosis*（knowledge）に由来．複数形は -gnoses となる．pro- は時間・順序に関して「前に（before）」の意の接頭辞．cf. diagnosis「診断」

Dictation
録音を聴いて空欄を埋め，各英文を完成させましょう．
① She did not (   ) first.
② She needed to live with the disorder (   ).
③ Rehabilitation (   ) of the disease.

Composition
日本語の意味に合うように〔　〕内の語（句）を並べ替えましょう．必要に応じて「,」を使用してください．
① この薬は癌患者の痛みを緩和するだろう．
　This〔 relieve, will, the pain, medicine, of, patients, cancer 〕.
② その政治家はその建物を復元してはどうかと提案した．
　The〔 that, suggested, be, the building, politician, restored 〕.
③ 研究所内での不注意はけがを招く可能性がある．
　Carelessness〔 in, result, laboratory, the, can, injuries, in 〕.
④ 彼女は持病を抱えて生きていくすべを身につけた．
　She〔 with, disease, learned, her, to, live, chronic 〕.
⑤ この薬は関節リウマチの進行を遅らせるために使用される．
　This〔 arthritis, rheumatoid, used, drug, progress, is, to, impede, the, of 〕.
⑥ 喫煙は肺がんになる危険性を高めることが知られている．
　It is known〔 smoking, that, risk, increases, lung, the, of, developing, cancer 〕.
⑦ 重度難聴の人は正常聴力の人よりも5倍認知症を発症しやすい．
　People〔 hearing loss, those, with, severe, are, five, likely to, times, more, develop, dementia, than, with 〕normal hearing.
⑧ 運動は健康増進と病気の予防において重要な役割を果たす．
　Physical〔 prevention, activity, plays, in, health, and, disease, a, critical, role, promotion 〕.
⑨ その計画は心臓病を減らすことをめざしている．
　The〔 at, heart, scheme, disease, is, reducing, aimed 〕.
⑩ その医療チームは医師，看護師，そして多くの他の医療専門家から構成されている．
　The medical〔 professionals, of, nurses, team, consists, and, doctors, many, other, healthcare 〕.

Medical Terms

第Ⅱ部のリスト（表1〜3）を参考に，空欄（1）〜（8）の後部連結形の意味を調べたうえで，例にならって空欄〔9〕〜〔15〕を埋めましょう．

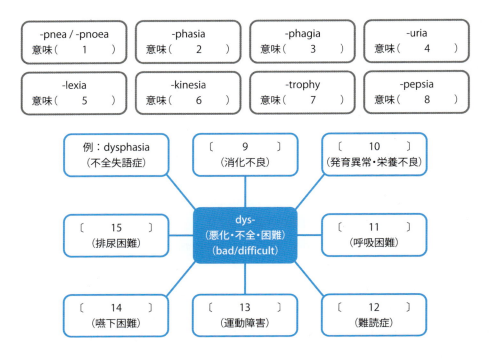

Let's try!

Make pairs and search for information about rheumatoid arthritis on the Web and share new information with your partner.

Unit 4

Colles' Fracture（コレス骨折）

　前腕には親指側を走る橈骨と小指側を走る尺骨の2本の骨があります．コレス骨折は転倒して手をついた際の衝撃により手首の関節に体重がかかることで橈骨が手首付近（遠位端）で折れる骨折を指します．骨折がひどい場合は，折れた橈骨の骨片が手の甲（手背）側にずれることにより，フォークを伏せたときのように弯曲してしまいます．また，骨折の程度により，痛み，腫れ，麻痺などの症状を伴います．なお，コレス骨折という名称はこの骨折の報告者であるアイルランドの外科医 Abraham Colles（1773-1843）に由来します．

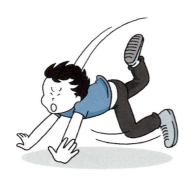
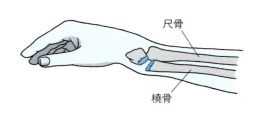

Reading 1

Vocabulary Study

以下の①〜⑩の語（句）の意味をa.〜j.から選びましょう．そのうえで実際に発音を練習してみましょう．

① break　　　　　　　　　a.（関節を）曲げる
② surface　　　　　　　　b. 楽天的な
③ deformed　　　　　　　c. 形が崩れた，変形した
④ fracture fragment　　　 d. 外面，表面
⑤ flexion　　　　　　　　 e. 骨片
⑥ extension　　　　　　　f. 衝撃を弱める
⑦ flex　　　　　　　　　　g. 掌，手のひら
⑧ palm　　　　　　　　　 h. 屈曲
⑨ prospect　　　　　　　 i. 見通し，予想，見込み
⑩ optimistic　　　　　　　j. 伸展

Unit 4 Colles' Fracture（コレス骨折）

Sakura Shirai is a 60-year-old woman living in Tsukuba City, Ibaraki. On a snowy day, Sakura went shopping at a nearby shopping mall. It was on her way to the shopping mall that the accident took place. She slipped and fell down on the hard surface of the sidewalk. As she quickly broke her fall with her outstretched arms, she didn't hit her head. However, she felt a sharp pain in her right hand which had hit the hard surface. It was clear that her right hand was fractured as it was deformed and looked like a dinner fork. So, she took a taxi from the site of the accident and hurried to the nearest orthopedic hospital.

The X-ray image of her right hand revealed a nearly-level fracture line at the distal end of the radius and a dorsal displacement of the fracture fragments. After studying the image carefully, her attending doctor reached the conclusion that the fracture would not heal correctly without a surgical procedure of the fragments, and performed an open reduction and internal fixation of the fractured wrist in which the fractured bone was put back into place and a locking plate was placed on the bone.

Takashi Yamada is an occupational therapist working for the hospital where Sakura underwent her operation. He was instructed by Sakura's attending doctor to start passive and active exercises for her on the day after surgery to prevent articular contracture of her hand. Takashi started her rehabilitation with the range of motion exercise of Sakura's interphalangeal joints securing her fractured wrist. He was extremely careful about flexion and extension exercises of her metacarpophalangeal joints so that Sakura would not feel pain. He asked Sakura to let him know when she felt pain during the exercise. Then, Takashi taught Sakura how to flex her wrist joint properly by herself. Takashi instructed her to support her right palm with her left palm and flex her injured right wrist back and forth slowly without using the strength of her left hand that supported the injured right hand. He also instructed her to relax her right hand.

After Sakura's rehabilitation, Takashi talked with her attending doctor about the prospect of her recovery and rehabilitation program. Takashi and the doctor talked about when to start training for grip strength and passive exercise of the wrist joint, and decided to wait until the formation of bony callus was confirmed on an X-ray image. The doctor explained that it would be about four weeks before she could start such exercises. The doctor also predicted that her muscle-strengthening exercises, which would enable her to use her right hand freely in her daily life, could probably be started in about eight weeks. The doctor was quite optimistic about Sakura's recovery and predicted that she would be free from limitation in the activities of daily living when the healing of the fracture was satisfactory.

Notes：break one's fall with〜 〜で転倒の衝撃を弱める，fracture line 骨折線，distal end of the radius/distal radius 橈骨遠位端，dorsal displacement of the fracture fragments 骨片の手背側へのずれ，open reduction and internal fixation 観血的整復固定術（皮膚を切開し，骨をプレート・スクリューなどで直接固定する方法），put back〜 into place 〜を元の位置に戻す，locking plate ロッキング・プレート，articular contracture 関節拘縮，interphalangeal joints 指節間関節，metacarpophalangeal joints 中手指節関節，bony callus 仮骨．

Reading Comprehension

本文の内容に一致するものにはT（True），異なるものにはF（False）を記入しましょう．

① Sakura broke her right hand on her way back from a nearby shopping mall.　（　）
② Sakura did not notice that her right hand was fractured at the site of the accident.　（　）
③ Sakura's attending doctor decided to perform an operation after studying the X-ray image of her right hand.　（　）
④ The doctor corrected the deformity of Sakura's right hand by using a locking plate.　（　）
⑤ Sakura's attending doctor told Takashi to start her rehabilitation a few weeks after the surgery.　（　）
⑥ Takashi was very careful about flexion and extension exercises so that Sakura would not feel pain.　（　）
⑦ Takashi talked with the doctor only at the beginning of Sakura's rehabilitation.　（　）
⑧ The X-ray image of Sakura's right hand failed to confirm the formation of bony callus.　（　）
⑨ Takashi and the doctor worked together to set up a rehabilitation program for Sakura.　（　）
⑩ The doctor was confident about the recovery of Sakura's right hand.　（　）

パーツと語源で覚える医学用語

● **interphalangeal** 指節間の
　inter-「間（between）」「相互に（mutually）」の意のラテン語由来の接頭辞と形容詞 phalangeal「指（節）骨の」からなり，「指節間の」の意の形容詞．

● **metacarpophalangeal** 中手指節の
　接頭辞 meta-「間（between）」＋前部連結形 carpo-「手根骨（carpus）」＋ phalangeal「指（節）骨の」からなり，「中手指節の」の意の形容詞．

Reading 2

Vocabulary Study

以下の①～⑩の語（句）の意味を a.～j. から選びましょう．そのうえで実際に発音を練習してみましょう．

① forearm   a. 特有な
② characteristic   b. 前腕
③ osteoporosis   c. 添え木，副子
④ external   d. 配置
⑤ prior   e. 固定する
⑥ alignment   f. 骨粗鬆症
⑦ splint   g. 外部（から）の
⑧ cast   h. 前の
⑨ immobilize   i. ギプス（包帯）
⑩ edema   j. 浮腫

　The Colles' fracture was named after Abraham Colles (1773-1843), an Irish surgeon, who first described this injury. It is a fracture of the distal radius in the forearm, or a break at the wrist end of the radius bone, with dorsal and radial displacement of the fractured bone, resulting in the characteristic "dinner fork" deformity, and is frequently accompanied by a fracture of the ulnar styloid.

　The fracture is common among post-menopausal elderly women who may be suffering from osteoporosis, which greatly increases the risk of fracture. Colles' fractures, however, can happen to younger people when they fall onto a hard surface and break their fall with outstretched arms or a radius bone is subjected to external force in an accident.

　There are many treatment options for distal radius fractures (DRFs), but the common goal is to enable the patient to attain his or her prior level of functioning. The doctor considers such factors as the nature of the fracture, the patient's age and activity level, and discusses with the patient about the best treatment option for his or her needs and wishes.

　Many DRFs can be treated conservatively. When the alignment of the fractured bone is out of place, the doctor realigns the broken bone fragments and corrects the deformity, which is a process called "reduction" technically. After the process of manipulative reduction, a splint or cast may be placed on the arm, and the injured wrist will be immobilized in palmar flexion and ulnar deviation for about five weeks. In the case in which the bone is splintered into three or more fragments, which is technically called comminuted fracture, or intra-articular injury which is too severe to be treated with manipulative reduction, surgery may be required to improve the alignment of the bone, and there are many ways of performing surgery. External fixation is utilized if necessary to assure rigid immobilization after surgery.

Most patients can return to their former activities after a DRF, but the degree of the injury, the kind of treatment, and the patient's response to the treatment all affect how quickly and to what extent the patient can recover. While the wrist is immobilized in a cast, passive and active exercises of the fingers are required at an early stage to prevent articular contracture of the fingers. Muscle strengthening exercises should be started with care after consulting the attending doctor after fracture healing has been confirmed and the cast has been removed. Therapists need to pay proper attention to edema, pain, scar formation and reflex sympathetic dystrophy caused by excessive exercise during rehabilitation.

> **Notes**: ulnar styloid 尺骨茎状突起, post-menopausal 閉経後の, ～is subjected to external force ～が外力を受ける, reduction 整復, manipulative reduction 徒手整復, palmar flexion and ulnar deviation 掌尺屈位（手首関節を小指側へ曲げながら掌側へ屈曲させた状態）, comminuted fracture 粉砕骨折, external fixation 創外固定, scar formation 瘢痕形成, reflex sympathetic dystrophy 反射性交感神経ジストロフィー.

Comprehension Questions

以下の問いに英語で答えましょう．

① What is the characteristic of the Colles' fracture?
② Who are prone to the Colles' fracture?
③ What is a typical case in which Colles' fractures happen to younger people?
④ What is the general goal in the treatment of distal radius fractures?
⑤ What does the doctor do first when the alignment of the fractured bone is out of place?
⑥ What is a comminuted fracture?
⑦ What is necessary if a fracture is too severe to be treated with manipulative reduction?
⑧ What factors affect the recovery from a DRF?
⑨ How should muscle strengthening exercises be started in the rehabilitation of DRFs?
⑩ What should therapists pay attention to during the rehabilitation of DRFs?

パーツと語源で覚える医学用語

● **post-menopausal**　閉経後の
　post-「後の（after, behind）」については Unit 1 を参照．menopausal「閉経期の」と結び付いて「閉経後の」の意．meno-「月経（menstruation）」はギリシャ語 *men*（month）に由来する前部連結形．meno- ＋ pause（休止）＝「閉経期の」．

● **osteoporosis**　骨粗鬆症
　oste(o)-「骨（bone）」については Unit 2 を参照．osteo- ＋ porosis「小孔形成，空洞形成」＝「骨粗鬆症」．poro- はギリシャ語 *poros*「細穴（pore）」に由来．ギリシャ語由来の接尾辞 -osis は「病的状態」の意．

● **intra-articular**　関節内の
　intra-「内の（within/inside）」＋ articular「関節の」＝「関節内の」．

● **dystrophy**　発育異常，栄養不良，ジストロフィー
　-trophy「栄養（nourishment）」はギリシャ語由来の後部連結形．dys-「悪化（bad）」＋ -trophy「栄養（nourishment）」＝「発育異常，栄養不良，ジストロフィー」．dys-「悪化（bad）」については Unit 3 を参照．

Dictation

録音を聴いて空欄を埋め，各英文を完成させましょう．

① Her right hand (   ).
② The doctor thought that (   ).
③ The Colles' fracture (   ) in the forearm
   (   ) of the fractured bone.

Composition

日本語の意味に合うように〔　〕内の語（句）を並べ替えましょう．必要に応じて「,」を使用してください．

① われわれは彼がその事故に対する責任があるという結論に達した．
   We〔 he, was, reached, responsible, the conclusion, that, for 〕the accident.
② サクラはリハビリを受けており，順調に回復中である．
   Sakura〔 is recovering, undergoing, has been, and, rehabilitation, steadily 〕.
③ その医者は彼女が日常生活活動において制約はなくなるだろうと予測した．
   The doctor〔 would, be free, activities, of, that, she, from, predicted, limitaion, in 〕daily living.
④ メアリーは部下に計画を実行するように指示した．
   Mary〔 the plan, out, instructed, her, to, carry, subordinates 〕.
⑤ 深刻な脳損傷の結果，広範囲にわたるケアとリハビリが必要になる可能性がある．
   Serious〔 brain, in, the need, for, extensive, injuries, can, result, care, and 〕rehabilitation.
⑥ 孤独と社会的孤立は高齢者にはよくあることだ．
   Loneliness〔 common, elderly, social, isolation, are, among, the, and 〕.
⑦ この情報により患者が自分のニーズに最適な病院を選ぶことが可能になるだろう．
   This information〔 best fit, the patients, to, choose, the hospitals, will, enable, that, their, needs 〕.
⑧ 専門家はその検査が，その病気からの回復が手遅れになる前に患者を早期に特定するかもしれないと話している．
   Experts say the test might〔 reverse, patients, early, late, to, it, before, identify, too, is 〕the illness.
⑨ その奨学金を受けるためにはどのような手続きが必要ですか．
   What〔 scholarship, process, receive, required, to, the, is 〕?
⑩ どの程度までその病院を信用してよいかわからない．
   I hardly〔 the, be, what, hospital, trusted, know, to, can, extent 〕.

Medical Terms

例にならって，以下のフローチャートの空欄を埋めましょう．

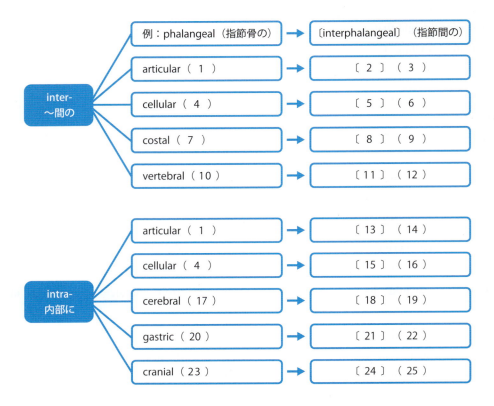

Let's try!

In pairs, discuss what you have learned about the Colles' fracture.

Unit 5

Locomotive Syndrome（ロコモティブシンドローム）

　ロコモティブシンドローム（運動器症候群）とは，日本整形外科学会が2007年に提唱した概念で，運動機能の障害による移動機能の低下した状態を表します．ロコモと略され，さまざまな運動器疾患（骨粗鬆症や変形性関節症など）や，加齢に伴う筋力低下，持久力低下などが原因で，要介護になるリスクが高い状態といわれています．超高齢社会を迎える日本では，ロコモの予防，早期発見，早期治療により，健康寿命を伸ばすことが喫緊の課題です．

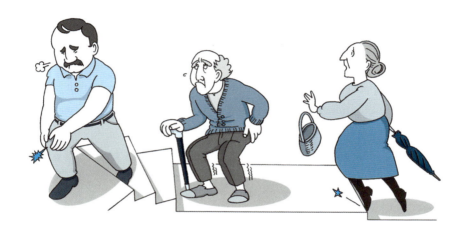

Reading 1

Vocabulary Study

以下の①〜⑩の語（句）の意味をa.〜j.から選びましょう．そのうえで実際に発音を練習してみましょう．

① pastime　　　　　　a. 多大な，途方もなく大きい
② diabetes　　　　　　b. ためらう
③ acute pain　　　　　c. 大学4年生
④ tremendous　　　　 d. 娯楽，気晴らし
⑤ health promotion　　e. 激痛
⑥ contribute　　　　　f.（〜するように）働きかける，励ます
⑦ encourage　　　　　g. 一因となる
⑧ hesitate　　　　　　h. 糖尿病
⑨ fit　　　　　　　　 i. 健康増進
⑩ senior　　　　　　　j. 健康な

Unit 5 Locomotive Syndrome（ロコモティブシンドローム）

Manabu Takagi is a 78-year-old man living in Yokohama. For approximately 40 years, he had been working as a salesman for one of the major department stores, and he retired 15 years ago. He now lives a free and easy life with his 75-year-old wife, Yuriko, who loves attending various activities to promote health.

Because he had never suffered from serious injuries or illnesses and had never been hospitalized, he believed that he was healthy. Above all, he was confident that walking around every day as a salesman had helped him to develop his strength. After retirement, however, having no favorite pastime in particular, he spent a lot of time lying on the sofa and watching television, without going for walks as before. As a result, he gained 10 kg in weight, and five years ago, he was diagnosed with diabetes.

After a while, it became harder for him to go upstairs, and his legs began to shake when he went up and down the stairs. In addition, he became slightly bowlegged. Last month, when he developed acute knee pain, he decided to see an orthopedist. He was diagnosed as having mild osteoarthritis of the knee. According to the doctor, the pain was partly because of his weight gain, which put tremendous stress on his knee muscles and joints. Therefore, he was told to perform knee muscle training and lose at least 5 kg.

A few days ago, he happened to watch a television program on health promotion, which introduced an easy way to check leg muscle strength. It was to put a sock on while standing on one leg. He tried it with his wife, Yuriko. However, far from being able to put a sock on, it was impossible for him to even stand on one leg. Yuriko, on the other hand, had no difficulty performing the task. The television program introduced a certain health condition called "locomotive syndrome" and mentioned that osteoarthritis was one of the main contributing diseases. Yuriko became concerned about Manabu's condition. She encouraged him to join the health promotion program for locomotive syndrome held in the community center near their house. At first, he hesitated to go, but he finally decided to join because taking part in the program seemed to be the reason why Yuriko was so fit.

Koichi Takagi, one of Mr. and Mrs. Takagi's grandsons, is a senior majoring in physical therapy. He was asked by the professor to help as a volunteer with the health promotion program for the elderly in the community center, as planned by the university. He had begun to work there only a month ago.

Yesterday, when Mr. and Mrs. Takagi visited the community center for the health promotion program, they were amazed to see their grandson Koichi working there as a volunteer. Koichi learned that locomotive syndrome could contribute to so-called "homeboundness," and he encouraged his grandparents to attend the program regularly. He is going to ask the professor to rearrange his work schedule so that he can work there once a week to help his grandparents.

Note：homeboundness（高齢者の）閉じこもり．

Reading Comprehension

本文の内容に一致するものにはT（True），異なるものにはF（False）を記入しましょう．

① After retirement, Manabu works at the community center as a volunteer.　（　　）

② Yuriko is too tired to attend various activities to promote health.　（　　）

③ Manabu was confident about his good health, because he had walked a lot every day for his job.　（　　）

④ Manabu had difficulty in going up and down the stairs.　（　　）

⑤ Manabu was hospitalized because the orthopedist diagnosed him as having osteoarthritis.　（　　）

⑥ Although Manabu had trouble putting a sock on while standing on one leg, it was easy for Yuriko to do so.　（　　）

⑦ Manabu decided not to take part in the health promotion program, because it did not look helpful for his health.　（　　）

⑧ Osteoarthritis is one of the causes of locomotive syndrome.　（　　）

⑨ Locomotive syndrome is one of the causes of homeboundness.　（　　）

⑩ Koichi is so busy studying that it is impossible for him to work at the community center to help his grandparents.　（　　）

パーツと語源で覚える医学用語

- **diabetes**　糖尿病（Unit 12を参照）

  サイフォン（siphon）を意味するギリシャ語 *diabetes* に由来．さらに遡ると，ギリシャ語 *diabainein*「通り過ぎる（go through）」にいたる．*dia-*「～を通って」+ *bainein*「行く」．

- **orthopedist/orthopaedist**　整形外科医（Unit 1, 3を参照）

  ortho-「まっすぐな，正しい」，-ist「～をする人，専門家，～主義者」．

- **osteoarthritis**　変形性関節症（骨関節炎）（Unit 2を参照）

  osteo-「骨」+ arthr-「関節」+ -itis「～炎」の構造．

- **locomotive syndrome**　ロコモティブシンドローム（運動器症候群）

  英語で運動器を locomotive organ と呼ぶことに由来．locomotive「運動の，運動性の」はラテン語 *locomotivus* に由来．*loco* は位置（position）を意味し，*loco-*「位置」+ *motive*「運動の」の構造．

  一方，syndrome「症候群」とはある病的状態において同時に発生する一群の症状のこと．ギリシャ語 *sundrome* に由来し，*sun-*「ともに」+ *dramein*「走る」の構造．

Reading 2

Vocabulary Study

以下の①～⑩の語（句）の意味を a.～j. から選びましょう．そのうえで実際に発音を練習してみましょう．

① healthy life expectancy　　a. 脳血管の
② internal organ　　　　　　 b. 有益な
③ cardiovascular　　　　　　 c. 椎骨
④ cerebrovascular　　　　　　d. 内臓
⑤ locomotive system　　　　　e. もろい
⑥ dysfunction　　　　　　　　f. 運動器系
⑦ brittle　　　　　　　　　　g. 心臓血管の
⑧ vertebra　　　　　　　　　 h. 機能障害
⑨ reinforce　　　　　　　　　i. 健康寿命
⑩ advantageous　　　　　　　 j. 強化する

　The three major factors that affect healthy life expectancy are dementia, metabolic syndrome, and locomotive syndrome. Metabolic syndrome is associated with disorders of the internal organs, including cardiovascular and cerebrovascular diseases. On the other hand, locomotive syndrome refers to problems associated with the locomotive system, including the muscles, bones, joints, cartilage, or the intervertebral discs. The function of the locomotive system is to support and move the body. Dysfunction of the locomotive system may restrict the ability to move. Therefore, in 2007, the Japanese Orthopedic Association proposed the concept of "locomotive syndrome" and defined it as a condition of having poor mobility requiring nursing care or being at risk of requiring nursing care.

　Locomotive syndrome develops due to two main causes. One cause is a disorder of the locomotive system itself, including osteoarthritis, osteoporosis, or spinal canal stenosis. These limit the joint range of motion, weaken muscle strength, and contribute to poor balance. The other cause is the dysfunction of the locomotive system due to aging. This limits the range of activity, leading to passiveness in daily lives, and resulting in "homeboundness." Musculoskeletal ambulation disability symptom complex (MADS) is one of the conditions included in locomotive syndrome and is associated with a particularly high risk of falls.

　One of the most hazardous problems associated with locomotive syndrome is the negative chain of the disorders. If an elderly individual with osteoporosis falls down, the risk of fracture is high because of brittle bones. Slipping and landing on the hands may cause a fracture of the wrist or a Colles' fracture. Falling down and hitting the waist can lead to fracture of the vertebrae including lumbar compression fractures. Falling down on the buttocks may twist the leg and cause a femoral neck fracture. These three fractures are of the greatest risk for the elderly.

To avoid such a negative chain, it is important not to miss the signs of locomotive syndrome and provide effective therapy in its early stages. Because maintaining the ability to stand up and sit down and walk independently are primary concerns, muscle training for the lower half of the body is the most recommended. Standing on one leg and doing simple squats, i.e., repeatedly standing up from a sitting position in a chair, are easy ways to improve balance and reinforce muscle strength. If patients are afraid of falling, they can lean onto or grab something to assist themselves. These two exercises are advantageous not only as therapy but also as preventive measures against locomotive syndrome, and they are easy to perform at home.

We are now facing a super-aged society. Everyone wants to have a healthy and active life as long as possible. Extending healthy life expectancy may depend on preventing diseases, such as locomotive syndrome. There are several warning signs of locomotive syndrome, for example, the inability to put on a sock while standing on one leg or slipping and stumbling in the home. Taking advantage of early recognition of these signs and taking preventive measures will help maintain independence and confidence.

> **Notes**: the intervertebral discs 椎間板, The Japanese Orthopedic Association 日本整形外科学会, spinal canal stenosis 脊柱管狭窄症, musculoskeletal ambulation disability symptom complex (MADS) 運動器不安定症. ロコモティブシンドロームより狭い概念で，65歳以上，日常生活自立度判定などの条件が加わる. **vertebrae** 椎骨（**vertebra** の複数形）, lumbar compression fracture 腰椎圧迫骨折.

Comprehension Questions

以下の問いに英語で答えましょう．

① What are the three major factors affecting healthy life expectancy?
② Who proposed the concept of locomotive syndrome?
③ According to the definition, what is locomotive syndrome?
④ What are two main causes of locomotive syndrome?
⑤ How does the disorder of the locomotive system affect the body?
⑥ How do elderly individuals with locomotive syndrome develop homeboundness?
⑦ What should we do to resolve the negative chain of locomotive syndrome?
⑧ What are two easy exercises to prevent locomotive syndrome?
⑨ What kind of society are we facing?
⑩ What are the typical warning signs of locomotive syndrome?

パーツと語源で覚える医学用語

- **cardiovascular** 心臓血管の
  cardi(o)-は「心臓」の意のギリシャ語由来の前部連結形．cardio-＋vascular「血管の」＝「心臓血管の」の意．vascul(o)-は「血管」の意のラテン語由来の前部連結形．

- **cerebrovascular** 脳血管の
  cerebr(o)-は「脳（brain）」の意のラテン語 *cerebrum* に由来する前部連結形．cerebro-＋vascular「血管の」＝「脳血管の」の意．

- **intervertebral** 椎間の
  inter-「間」＋vertebral「脊椎（骨）の」＝「椎間の」の意．Unit 4 の interphalangeal の解説および Medical Terms を参照．

- **spinal** 脊柱の
  spin(o)-「脊柱」はラテン語由来の前部連結形．同じくラテン語由来の接尾辞 -al「〜の」と連結して形容詞をつくる．

- **stenosis** 狭窄症
  sten(o)-は「狭い（narrow）」の意のギリシャ語由来の前部連結形．-osis は「病的状態」を表すギリシャ語由来の接尾辞．

- **dysfunction** 機能障害
  Unit 3 を参照．

- **musculoskeletal** 筋骨格の
  muscul(o)-は「筋（muscle）」の意のラテン語由来の前部連結形．musculo-＋skeletal「骨格の」＝「筋骨格の」の意．skelet(o)-は「骨格（skeleton）」の意のラテン語由来の前部連結形．

- **osteoporosis** 骨粗鬆症
  Unit 4 を参照．

Dictation

録音を聴いて空欄を埋め，各英文を完成させましょう．

① The Japanese Orthopedic Association (

) requiring nursing care.

② If an elderly person falls down,( ).

③ These two exercises are ( )

against locomotive syndrome.

Composition

日本語の意味に合うように〔 〕内の語（句）を並べ替えましょう．必要に応じて「，」を使用してください．

① 彼は健康には自信があり，100歳まで生きると言っている．

He says that 〔 confident, he is, live, and will, 100 years old, of his health, to be 〕.

② 異常がないどころか，彼は糖尿病だと診断された．

Far from being fine,〔 was, diabetes, diagnosed, as, he, having 〕.

③ 私の祖母は手すりにつかまらずに階段をのぼるのは大変そうだ．

My grandmother 〔 to have difficulty, up the stairs, seems, in, holding onto, climbing, without 〕 the handrail.

④ 変形性関節症は，運動機能系にかかわる疾患のひとつである．

Osteoarthritis is 〔 the diseases, the locomotive system, associated, one of, with 〕.

⑤ 理学療法士はさまざまな運動療法を利用し，一人で歩くよう祖父を励ました．

The physical therapist〔 my grandfather, to walk, kinesiotherapy, encouraged, by himself, using, various types of 〕.

⑥ 整形外科学会によると，その疾患は介護を必要とする運動機能の障害と定義されている．

The Orthopedic Association 〔 the locomotive system, a disorder, the disease, defines, nursing care, as, of, requiring 〕.

⑦ 加齢が原因で，祖母は長時間歩くことが難しくなってきている．

My grandmother 〔 aging, trouble, has had, for a long time, walking, due to 〕.

⑧ 一番大事なことは，適度な運動とバランスのとれた食事である．

What is 〔 is, exercise, and a balanced diet, moderate, most important 〕.

⑨ 健康寿命を伸ばすには，日常生活での前向きな態度が肝要だ．

We should 〔 to extend, have, a positive, healthy life expectancy, our daily life, attitude, in 〕.

⑩ 祖父は私の助言で診察を受ける決心をした．

My grandfather 〔 my advice, up, to see, a doctor, made, on, his mind 〕.

Medical Terms

第Ⅱ部のリスト（表1〜3）を参考に，下記の語彙パーツを組み合わせて①〜⑩の医学用語をつくりましょう．必要があれば同じパーツを何度使ってもかまいません．

cardi(o)-	cerebr(o)-	skelet(o)-	pulmon(o)-
muscul(o)-	spin(o)-	vascul(o)-	angi(o)-
scler(o)-	arteri(o)-	sten(o)-	
-al	-ar	-ary	-osis

① 肺塞栓症：(　　　　　) embolism
② 脳血管系：(　　　　　) system
③ 心臓血管系：(　　　　　) system
④ 心肺蘇生法：(　　　　　) resuscitation
⑤ 脳脊髄液：(　　　　　) fluid
⑥ 血管狭窄：(　　　　　)
⑦ 動脈狭窄：(　　　　　)
⑧ 動脈硬化：(　　　　　)
⑨ 多発性硬化症：multiple (　　　　　)
⑩ 筋骨格系：(　　　　　) system

Let's try!

　　The Japanese Orthopedic Association has introduced seven warning signs of locomotive syndrome. Look up what the signs are and check to see if you and your partner have any.

Unit 6

Chronic Lower Back Pain （慢性腰痛症）

　成人の70％が生涯に一度は腰痛を経験すると言われています．痛みが続く長さによって，「急性腰痛」と「慢性腰痛」に分けられますが，痛みの大きさや範囲はさまざまで，原因が明確でないものもあります．日常生活のなかで頻発する疾患ですが，超高齢社会となる日本では，老老介護といった社会現象のなかで，介護現場での慢性腰痛が大きな問題となっています．

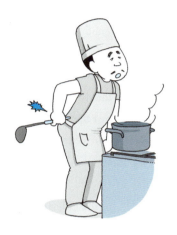
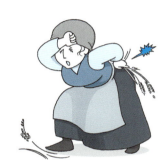

Reading 1

Vocabulary Study

以下の①～⑩の語（句）の意味を a.～j. から選びましょう．そのうえで実際に発音を練習してみましょう．

① junior college　　　　　a. 産休
② share　　　　　　　　　b. 仕事量
③ intensive　　　　　　　 c. 集中的な
④ transferring　　　　　　d. その後の
⑤ maternity leave　　　　 e. 短大
⑥ workload　　　　　　　 f. 身体機能
⑦ physical function　　　 g. 移乗，身体移動
⑧ flexibility　　　　　　　h. 再発率
⑨ subsequent　　　　　　 i. 分担する
⑩ recurrence rate　　　　 j. 柔軟性

Mari Takada is a 35-year-old woman who works as a care worker at a nursing home in Utsunomiya, Tochigi Prefecture. She began working as a care worker after she graduated from junior college. She married seven years ago and has a 6-year-old son and a 4-year-old daughter. Because her husband Satoshi also works as a care worker, he understands that she is busy working as well as raising their children. Therefore, they share the housework.

Because she is one of the most experienced workers, Mari is in charge of various assistance activities for the nursing home residents who need intensive care. These assistance activities include bathing, toileting, and transferring. Mari, therefore, occasionally experienced back pain but every time she experienced pain, it disappeared in a few days. Three months ago, after one of the other staff members went on maternity leave, however, Mari's workload increased even more and the back pain worsened and lasted for longer periods of time. Eventually, she visited an orthopedic clinic and was diagnosed with chronic lower back pain. Under the guidance of the doctor, she began rehabilitation.

Yoshiko Noguchi is a physical therapist at the clinic. She evaluated Mari's physical function and noticed that the strength of the trunk expansion muscles, the endurance of the muscles, and the flexibility of the muscles around the hip joint had decreased. Yoshiko confirmed that the pain became more severe in a bending position. Magnetic resonance imaging (MRI) showed atrophy of the multifidus muscles. Yoshiko instructed Mari how to train the trunk expansion muscles and how to improve the flexibility of the muscles around the hip joint. She recommended that basic muscle training and stretching of the back muscles and the muscles around the hip joint would be most effective. She also instructed Mari how to move her body without overloading it when she was performing assistance activities for the elderly.

Mari performed these therapeutic exercises at home every evening and she visited the clinic once a week for rehabilitation. She initially thought that her two children would complain about her therapy because it would shorten the important time that the children spent with their mother. Unexpectedly, however, they were glad to help with her exercises by supporting her hands and legs, and this greatly reduced her stress. Therefore, by three weeks, her lower back pain had been relieved.

A subsequent physical examination revealed improvement in the strength of the trunk expansion muscles and endurance of the muscles. Although Mari was considerably pleased with the result, Yoshiko advised her to continue the stretching exercises after work because lower back pain has a high recurrence rate.

Notes: trunk expansion muscle 体幹伸展筋, endurance of the muscles 筋持久力, bending position 前屈姿勢, atrophy of the multifidus muscles 多裂筋の萎縮.

Reading Comprehension

本文の内容に一致するものには T（True），異なるものには F（False）を記入しましょう．

① Mari lives in Utsunomiya with her husband and two sons. （　　）
② Mari works as a care worker at a nursing home. （　　）
③ Although Mari has a lot of experience as a care worker, she is not required to do responsible jobs. （　　）
④ Mari's back worsened because her husband did not help with the housework. （　　）
⑤ Mari was diagnosed with lower back pain and began rehabilitation. （　　）
⑥ Yoshiko evaluated that the flexibility of Mari's muscles was inadequate. （　　）
⑦ Yoshiko advised Mari to stop working and to rest at home. （　　）
⑧ Mari was able to do therapeutic exercises every evening with the support of her children. （　　）
⑨ Despite therapeutic exercises, the physical examination after three weeks did not show any improvement of Mari's muscle condition. （　　）
⑩ Mari was advised to continue therapeutic exercises in order to prevent the recurrence of lower back pain. （　　）

パーツと語源で覚える医学用語

● **orthopedic** 整形外科の
orth(o)- は「まっすぐな (straight)，正しい (right, correct)」の意のギリシャ語 *orthos* (straight, right) が語源．Unit 1 を参照．

● **atrophy** 萎縮
a-/an- は「無・不・非 (not/without)」の意のギリシャ語由来の接頭辞．-trophy は「栄養 (nourishment)，成長 (growth)」の意のギリシャ語由来の後部連結形．

● **diagnose** 診断する
接頭辞 dia-「離れて」+ -gnosis「認識」= diagnosis「診断」．Unit 3 を参照．

● **overload** 負担をかけすぎる
接頭辞 over「過剰に (excessively)」+ load「負わせる」=「負担をかけすぎる」．

● **recurrence** 再発
ラテン語 *recurrere*（戻る）に由来．re-「再び (again)，戻って (back)」+ *currere*「走る (run)」．

Reading 2

Vocabulary Study

以下の①〜⑩の語（句）の意味を a. 〜 j. から選びましょう．そのうえで実際に発音を練習してみましょう．

① subjective symptom   a. 解決する
② strained back   b. 提供
③ resolve   c. 過剰な
④ dull   d. 自覚症状
⑤ trigger   e. きっかけとなる
⑥ underlie   f. 姿勢
⑦ posture   g. 基礎となる
⑧ provision   h. ぎっくり腰
⑨ coping skill   i. （痛みが）鈍い
⑩ excessive   j. 対応能力

Lumbago or lower back pain is quite common, and it has been reported that more than 70 percent of all adults experience lower back pain at some time in their lives. Therefore, the number of individuals with subjective symptoms of lower back pain is also high.

Lower back pain can be divided into two types: acute and chronic. Acute lower back pain is characterized by an acute, sharp, and severe pain, which can prevent movement. It can be caused by injuries, accidents, or sudden shock to the back from one simple movement, such as reaching for something. A strained back is one of the most common causes of acute lower back pain. Although the pain is strong, with quiet rest, it improves day-by-day and eventually resolves completely. Almost 90 percent of acute lower back pain is said to be resolved within one month.

On the other hand, lower back pain that lasts for more than three months is called chronic lower back pain. The pain itself is not as sharp as acute lower back pain, but it is dull and lasts longer, and it is almost impossible to cure completely. In some cases, the source of the pain is not clear, and even if the condition or the injury that triggered the pain is resolved completely, the pain will continue to bother the patient.

Whether the lower back pain is acute or chronic, if the exact cause of the pain can be defined, it is referred to as specific lower back pain. Typical examples of specific lower back pain are lumbar disc herniation, lumbar spinal canal stenosis, and lumbar compression fractures. Each specific cause should be treated differently according to the diagnosis. However, about 85 percent of lower back pain is non-specific, indicating that the exact cause or the exact source of the pain cannot be identified on X-ray, computed tomography (CT), or MRI, even if the patient is in pain. In these cases, the pain may originate from multiple causes, such as physical damage, the effects of long-term incorrect posture, stress, etc.

Therefore, the treatment of non-specific lower back pain includes different general categories, such as rehabilitation, medication, and the provision of coping skills. Typical rehabilitation involves therapeutic exercises, such as stretching of the back muscles and the muscles around the hip joint to strengthen the muscles of the trunk and lower limbs. Although these exercises may reduce pain and improve quality of life (QOL), the additional provision of coping skills in order to manage daily activities without excessive stress is essential.

In a super-aged society, such as that of Japan, lower back pain caused by adopting a bending position while caring for the elderly is not only an individual physical problem but also one of the most serious social problems, especially in the elder-to-elder nursing conditions. This problem cannot be solved without changing the ways in which care work is carried out and reducing the burden of care work. The Ministry of Health, Labour and Welfare has suggested ways to lighten the physical burden of conventional care work by using various types of machinery. Such procedures may be key factors in reducing chronic lower back pain.

Notes: lumbago 腰痛, **specific lower back pain** 特異的腰痛, **non-specific** 非特異的, **lumbar disc herniation** 椎間板ヘルニア, **lumbar spinal canal stenosis** 腰部脊柱管狭窄症, **elder-to-elder nursing** 老老介護.

Comprehension Questions
以下の問いに英語で答えましょう．
① What percentage of adults are reported to experience lower back pain?
② What is the main feature of acute lower back pain?
③ How does chronic lower back pain differ from acute lower back pain?
④ What is the difference between specific lower back pain and non-specific lower back pain?
⑤ What are typical examples of specific lower back pain?
⑥ Why does non-specific lower back pain require various treatments?
⑦ What kind of rehabilitation is required for non-specific lower back pain?
⑧ Apart from rehabilitation, what is necessary to improve the QOL of lower back pain patients?
⑨ Why is lower back pain one of the greatest social problems in Japan?
⑩ What does the Ministry of Health, Labour and Welfare suggest in order to reduce the burden of care work?

パーツと語源で覚える医学用語

● **lumbago** 腰痛
前部連結形 lumb(o)-「腰（loin），腰椎と～との」はラテン語 *lumbus*（loin）に由来．

● **arthropathy** 関節症，関節疾患
-pathy は「病気（disease）」や「療法（treatment）」の意のギリシャ語由来の後部連結形．
arthr(o)-「関節（joint）」に結び付いて関節疾患の意．

● **lumbar** 腰の
連結形 lumb(o)-「腰（loin），腰椎と～との」+接尾辞 -ar「～の」=「腰の」．

● **spinal canal stenosis** 脊柱管狭窄症
spin(o)- は「脊柱」，sten(o)- は「狭い（narrow）」，-osis は「病的状態」の意．Unit 5 の spinal, stenosis を参照．

● **diagnosis** 診断
接頭辞 dia-「離れて」+-gnosis「認識」= diagnosis「診断」．-gnosis は「知識（knowledge）・認識（recognition）」の意の後部連結形．ギリシャ語 *gnosis*（knowledge）に由来．Unit 3, diagnose を参照．

● **tomography** 断層撮影
tomo-「切断（cut）」+-graphy「写法・記録法」=「断層撮影」．tomo-, -graphy ともにギリシャ語由来の連結形．

Dictation

録音を聴いて空欄を埋め，各英文を完成させましょう．

① Her workload （　　　　　　　　　　　　　　　　　　　　　　　）．

② Acute lower back pain （　　　　　　　　　　　　　　　　　　　）．

③ （　　　　　　　　　　　　　　　　　） lower back pain．

Composition

日本語の意味に合うように〔　〕内の語（句）を並べ替えましょう．必要に応じて「,」を使用してください．

① 彼はいつもアルバイトで忙しそうだ．

He always 〔 working, looks, part-time, busy 〕．

② 私の祖父は入浴，排泄に助けが必要である．

My grandfather 〔 bathing, assitance, in, needs, and toileting 〕．

③ 彼の腰痛は3ヵ月続いたので，整形外科を受診した．

He visited 〔 for three months, since, lasted, his back pain, an orthopedic clinic 〕．

④ 体力検査によると，股関節の柔軟性が衰えていることがわかった．

The physical examination 〔 that, had decreased, the flexibility, showed, of the muscles around the hip joints 〕．

⑤ 彼女は喜んで母の脚を支えて運動を手助けした．

She was 〔 with, help, her mother's exercise, glad to, supporting her legs, by 〕．

⑥ 腰痛の自覚症状のある人の数は増加している．

The 〔 subjective symptoms, number, of, with, individuals, of lower back pain 〕 is increasing.

⑦ 痛みを引き起こしたけがが治癒したにもかかわらず，痛みは相変わらず彼を苦しめている．

Although 〔 triggered, the injury, the pain, that, resolved 〕, the pain continues to bother him.

⑧ 痛みが強かろうが弱かろうが，その原因をはっきりさせなければならない．

The exact cause of the pain 〔 whether, is, identified, should be, or weak, the pain, strong 〕．

⑨ 高齢者介護の際に腰を曲げた姿勢を続けることは腰痛の一大原因である．

Adopting 〔 while, is, a bending position, the elderly, caring for 〕 one of the biggest causes of lower back pain.

⑩ 介護の負担を減らすことなしに介護者不足を解決することはできない．

The shortage of 〔 solved, caregivers, the burden, without, reducing, cannot be 〕 of care work.

Medical Terms

第Ⅱ部のリスト（表1～3）を参考に，下記の語彙パーツを組み合わせて①～⑦の医学用語をつくりましょう．必要があれば同じパーツを何度使ってもかまいません．

| dys- | eu- | hyper- | a- |
| leuk(o)- | oste(o)- | neur(o)- | my(o)- |
| -trophy |

① 栄養障害，発育異常：（　　　　　）
② 萎縮：（　　　　　）
③ 肥大：（　　　　　）
④ 栄養良好：（　　　　　）
⑤ 骨栄養：（　　　　　）
⑥ 白質ジストロフィー/白質萎縮症：（　　　　　）
⑦ 神経栄養：（　　　　　）

Let's try!

Choose an example of care work and think of ways to lighten the physical burden of the work. Then, exchange your ideas with your partners.

Unit 7

Spinal Cord Injury（脊髄損傷）

　脊髄は，脳と体の各部を結ぶ重要な通信経路であり，知覚および運動の刺激伝達を行い，反射機能をつかさどっています．脊髄は神経索で，脊柱管内に位置しています．強力な外力が加わり脊椎の脱臼骨折があると，脊髄に圧迫や挫創が起こり，脊髄が損傷されます．受傷者ができるだけ多くの機能を回復するためには，リハビリテーションが必要です．

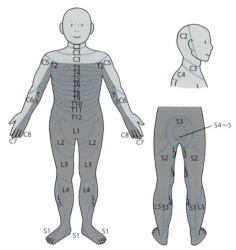

第6頸髄神経まで残存した脊髄損傷患者の感覚障害領域

Reading 1

Vocabulary Study

以下の①〜⑩の語（句）の意味をa.〜j.から選びましょう．そのうえで実際に発音を練習してみましょう．

① spinal　　　　　　　　　a. 四肢麻痺
② forward dislocation　　　b. 再生の
③ cervical　　　　　　　　c. 共感する
④ anterior　　　　　　　　d. 屈曲の
⑤ reposition　　　　　　　e. 脊髄の
⑥ quadriplegia　　　　　　f. 自助具
⑦ empathize　　　　　　　g. 前の，頭部に近い
⑧ regenerative　　　　　　h. 頸部の
⑨ flexural　　　　　　　　i. 整復させる
⑩ self-help device　　　　　j. 前方脱臼

Koji Chiba is a third-year university student. While he was enjoying himself at the seaside during his summer vacation last month, he had a diving accident and passed out. His friend, who had immediately noticed, saved him and took him to the hospital. The doctor found that he had forward dislocation of the sixth cervical vertebra (Figure 1).

After having anterior spinal fusion of the cervical spine, Koji started passive joint exercise and gradually worked on a muscle-strengthening program. His bone was repositioned by surgery (Figure 2), but the damage to the spinal nerves was so severe that he had lost almost all muscular strength and nerve sensation of the seventh cervical vertebra and below, and his recovery did not seem possible. He was diagnosed with severe quadriplegia.

An occupational therapist, Takako Haneda, is 25 years old, near Koji's age. She started Koji on a push-up exercise program. He told her that his arms and legs would not recover. He added that his doctor had told him that he would not be able to walk again. She understood his concern and remained silent for a while.

Takako empathized with Koji, who had become quadriplegic after the sudden accident and could not walk by himself. However, she knew that no matter how much she sympathized with him, neither his symptoms nor his worries would disappear.

When Takako asked Koji if he was troubled by the fact that he would not be able to walk again, he replied that broken spinal nerves do not recover. He added that he knew it was no use regretting what had happened. She nodded slowly and asked him whether he would feel better if he could manage to move by himself. He answered that it might make him feel better to some extent but also said that he found it difficult to accept the harsh reality. Takako thought that using a robot suit or having his spinal cord reproduced by regenerative medicine might enable him to walk again, but she did not say that.

Koji and Takako resumed the push-up exercises. He was able to move the pectoralis major and serratus anterior, so he was able to pull his upper extremities toward his trunk. He would eventually be able to transfer to a wheelchair alone. He did not have flexural muscular strength in his fingers, but he would be able to grasp an object with a self-help device and functional tenodesis-like action and acquire independent skills for activities of daily living (ADL) after some time. He will go back to the university in a wheelchair in several months and start to plan his senior thesis and consider his future occupation.

Notes：**anterior spinal fusion（surgery）** 頸椎前方固定術，**pectoralis major** 大胸筋，**serratus anterior** 前鋸筋，**tenodesis-like action** 腱固定作用.

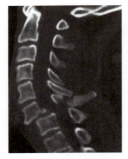

Figure 1. 第6頸椎の脱臼骨折

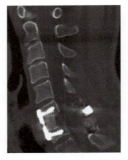

Figure 2. 頸椎の修復固定術後

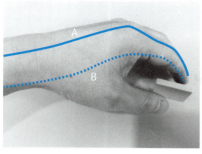 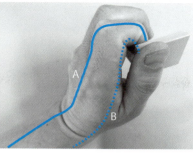

第6頸椎損傷患者は手指の屈曲は不能で，物をつまむことは困難．手関節の背屈はできる．
① 手関節が掌屈すると手指伸筋 (A) が緊張して手指は伸びる．
② 手関節が背屈すると手指屈筋 (B) は緊張して手指は曲がる．
この作用は手指屈筋を短縮させる外科手術で強くできるが，手指屈筋の自然短縮でも得られる．

Figure 3. Tenodesis（腱固定）を利用した把持動作

Reading Comprehension

本文の内容に一致するものにはT（True），異なるものにはF（False）を記入しましょう．

① Koji had an accident when he was driving. （　）
② Koji was taken to the hospital by his family. （　）
③ Koji had forward dislocation of a cervical vertebra. （　）
④ Koji had surgery which adjusted the position of his bone. （　）
⑤ Koji has had paralysis of all four limbs. （　）
⑥ Takako said that Koji's arms and legs would recover in the future. （　）
⑦ Koji thinks that it is important to reflect on what has happened. （　）
⑧ Koji said that he would probably feel better if he could move by himself. （　）
⑨ Takako told Koji that he might be able to walk if he uses a robot suit or has his spinal cord reproduced. （　）
⑩ Koji has independent ADL skills and is thinking about his future occupation. （　）

パーツと語源で覚える医学用語

● **cervical** 頸部の
　cervic(o)- は「首（neck），頸部（cervix）」の意のラテン語由来の前部連結形．子宮頸管部を指す場合もある．

● **quadriplegia/tetraplegia** 四肢麻痺
　-plegia は「麻痺（paralysis）」の意のギリシャ語由来の後部連結形．quadri- は「4」の意のラテン語由来の前部連結形．ギリシャ語系の前部連結形 tetra-「4」と連結しても同じ意味．

● **tenodesis** 腱固定
　teno- は「腱（tendon）」の意のギリシャ語由来の前部連結形．-desis は「束縛（binding），固定（fixation）」の意のギリシャ語由来の後部連結形．

Reading 2

Vocabulary Study

以下の①～⑩の語（句）の意味を a.～j. から選びましょう．そのうえで実際に発音を練習してみましょう．

① neurotransmission		a. 人工呼吸装置	
② necrosis		b. 対麻痺	
③ paralysis		c. 最小限にする	
④ paraplegia		d. 安定させる	
⑤ approximately		e. 麻痺	
⑥ stabilize		f. 体位の，姿勢の	
⑦ minimize		g. 壊死	
⑧ respirator		h. 拘縮	
⑨ postural		i. 神経伝達	
⑩ contracture		j. およそ	

　An injury of the spinal cord causes motor paralysis and sensory impairment in the damaged part and below because the neurotransmission pathway from the brain to the body is disturbed. If there is necrosis in the spinal cord even locally, recovery cannot be expected, and complete or incomplete paralysis remains depending on the degree of injury of the spinal cord and nerve roots. It is likely that cervical cord injury will lead to quadriplegia, thoracic cord injury will cause paraplegia, and lumbosacral spinal cord and cauda equina injury will result in flaccid paraplegia. This causal relationship is well known.

　The frequency of spinal cord injury in Japan is approximately 40 persons per million, and around 4,000 persons incur spinal cord injury every year. Approximately 70 percent of these suffer from cervical spinal cord injury. The most common cause is traffic accidents, which comprise 40 percent of cases. The spinal cord injury rate among men is approximately four times as high as that among women.

　In the acute stage of spinal cord injury, the condition of the whole body should be stabilized and the damage to nerves should be minimized. Treatments include medication and surgery to relieve pressure on the spinal cord. Cervical spinal cord injury and higher thoracic spinal cord injury can impair lung function and might require the use of a respirator.

　Unfortunately it is difficult, if not impossible, to completely cure spinal cord injuries in modern medicine. Therefore, the aim of post-acute treatment is not to restore physical function to its state before the spinal cord injury but to train the body and enhance the degree of independence in everyday life.

　The rehabilitation program includes postural change, respiration training, and range-of-motion exercises to prevent articular contracture. An active rehabilitation program can be started when the patient's physical condition becomes stable. The impairment caused by spinal cord injury depends to some extent on which part of the spinal cord is damaged. Predicting residual abilities can help in the determination of the most appropriate exercise program. For example, paraplegic patients need muscular strength to lift their body and propel the wheelchair. The push-up exercise is fundamental training for moving on the bed and the floor with the power of the upper limbs（Figure 4）. Persons with quadriplegia need flexibility of the hip joints to move on the floor with their arms and change their clothes. Muscular training and range-of-motion exercises for the joints should be well planned and performed.

Notes: thoracic cord injury 胸髄損傷, lumbosacral spinal cord 腰仙髄, cauda equina 馬尾神経, flaccid paraplegia 弛緩性対麻痺.

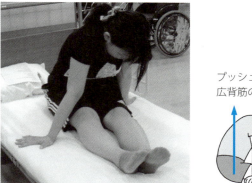

Figure 4．脊髄損傷患者のプッシュアップ練習

Comprehension Questions

以下の問いに英語で答えましょう．

① What does an injury of the spinal cord lead to?
② What is likely to cause quadriplegia?
③ What may result in flaccid paraplegia?
④ How many people incur spinal cord injury every year?
⑤ What is the most common cause of spinal cord injury?
⑥ What is important for the body in the acute stage of spinal cord injury?
⑦ Why might a respirator be required for cervical spinal cord injury and higher thoracic spinal cord injury?
⑧ What is the aim of post-acute treatment?
⑨ When can the patient with spinal cord injury start an active rehabilitation program?
⑩ What do paraplegic patients build muscular strength for?

パーツと語源で覚える医学用語

● **paralysis** 麻痺
ギリシャ語 *paraluein*「一方の側でゆるめる」に由来．*para-*「側で（beside）」+ *luein*「ゆるめる（loosen）」の構造．para- は「側で（beside）」の意の接頭辞．-lysis は「分解（decomposition），溶解（dissolution），分離（detachment）」の意の後部連結形．

● **thoracic** 胸部の
thorac(o)- は「胸（thorax/chest）」の意のギリシャ語由来の前部連結形．-ic は形容詞をつくる接尾辞．

● **paraplegia** 対麻痺（ついまひ）（脊髄の病気・傷害に起因する両下肢の麻痺）
元来は体の全体あるいは一部の麻痺を指して用いられたが，後に両下肢や体幹の麻痺を指して用いられるようになった．ギリシャ語 *paraplessein*「片側の一撃」に由来．para-「側（に）」+ -plegia「麻痺」の構造．後部連結形 -plegia「麻痺（paralysis）」は「一打（strike）」の意のギリシャ語 *plege* に由来．

● **lumbosacral** 腰仙の
lumb(o)- は「腰（loin）」の意のラテン語由来の前部連結形．sacral は「仙骨の，仙椎の」の意の形容詞．sacr(o)- は「仙骨（sacrum）」の意のラテン語由来の前部連結形．前部連結形を2つ含む lumbo- + sacr- + -al という構造になる．

Dictation

録音を聴いて空欄を埋め，各英文を完成させましょう．

① The patient lost almost all (　　　　　　　　　　　　　　　　　) of the seventh cervical vertebra and below.

② If there is necrosis in the spinal cord even locally, recovery cannot be expected, and (　　　　　　　　　　　　　　　　).

③ Persons with quadriplegia need (　　　　　　　　　　　　　　　　　) to move on the floor with their arms and change their clothes.

Composition

日本語の意味に合うように〔　〕内の語（句）を並べ替えましょう．必要に応じて「,」を使用してください．

① 医師は患者に第5頸椎が脱臼していると告げた．
The doctor 〔 the patient, cervical vertebra, dislocation, the fifth, that, had, told, he, of 〕.

② 再生医療で脊髄が再生できれば，その選手はまた走れるかもしれない．
The athlete might 〔 medicine, again, his spinal, be, run, reproduced, cord, regenerative, able to, he has, if, by 〕.

③ その患者は手指の屈曲筋力はないが，自助具で物の把握が可能である．
Although the patient does not have flexural muscular 〔 she, object, device, grasp, with, her fingers, can, strength, self-help, in, a, an 〕.

④ 過半数の脊髄損傷受傷者は頸髄損傷である．
More than half of the persons 〔 cord, suffer, injury, who, from, spinal, incur 〕 cervical spinal cord injury.

⑤ 男性の脊髄損傷の割合は女性よりもおよそ4倍高い．
The spinal cord injury rate among men 〔 times, as, four, as, is, high, approximately 〕 that among women.

⑥ 治療には脊髄の圧迫を緩和する手術が含まれる．
Treatments 〔 relieve, cord, surgery, the spinal, on, pressure, include, to 〕.

⑦ 急性期後の治療の目標は，身体のトレーニングを行い日常生活の自立度を上げることである．
The aim of 〔 treatment, to, enhance, the degree, the body, post-acute, and, is, train 〕 of independence in everyday life.

⑧ 患者の身体の状態が安定したら，積極的なリハビリテーションプログラムが開始できる．
An active rehabilitation program 〔 when, stable, condition, started, the patient's, be, becomes, physical, can 〕.

⑨ プッシュアップの練習は，上肢の力で移動するための基本的なトレーニングである．
The push-up exercise is 〔 the upper, the power, for, training, limbs, moving, with, fundamental, of 〕.

⑩ 筋力トレーニングと関節可動域の訓練は，しっかり計画され実行された．
Muscular training and 〔 performed, for, well planned, the joints, range-of-motion, and, were, exercises 〕.

Medical Terms

（A）第Ⅱ部のリスト（表1～3）や辞書を参考に，空欄（1）～（8）の接辞や連結形の意味を調べたうえで，例にならって空欄〔9〕～〔15〕を埋めましょう．

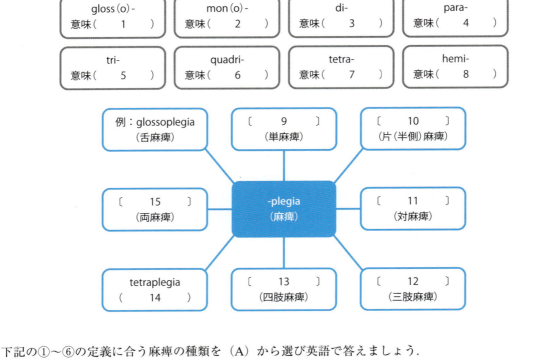

下記の①～⑥の定義に合う麻痺の種類を（A）から選び英語で答えましょう．
① 体の片側の麻痺．　　　　　　　　　　　　　　　（　　　　　　　　　　）
② 片側の上下肢と反対側の一肢の麻痺．　　　　　　（　　　　　　　　　　）
③ 四肢すべての麻痺．　　　　　　　　　　　　　　（　　　　　／　　　　）
④ 左右の脚・腕のうち，一肢だけに起こる麻痺．　　（　　　　　　　　　　）
⑤ 両下肢の麻痺．典型的には脊髄損傷により起こる．（　　　　　　　　　　）
⑥ 体の両側の対応する部分の麻痺．典型的には腕よりも足の麻痺が激しい．
　　　　　　　　　　　　　　　　　　　　　　　　（　　　　　　　　　　）

Let's try!

What can cause spinal cord injury? Discuss the question in groups.

Unit 8

Adjustment Disorder and Symptomatic Depression
（適応障害と症候性うつ状態）

　適応障害は，ある社会環境においてうまく適応することができず，さまざまな心身の症状を呈する症候群です．ある特定の状況や出来事が，その人にとってとてもつらく耐えがたく感じられ，そのために気分や行動面に多様な症状が現れるものです．たとえば憂うつな気分や不安感が強くなり，涙もろくなったり，過剰に心配したり，神経が過敏になったりします．また，頭痛，不眠，食欲不振，腹痛などの身体症状，遅刻，欠勤，過剰飲酒などの問題行動がみられることもあります．そして，対人関係，社会的機能が不良となり，引きこもってうつ状態となる場合もあります．

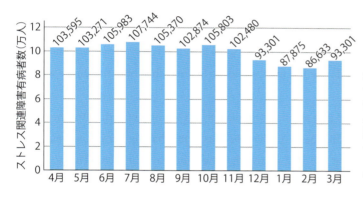

うつ・適応障害を含む，ストレス関連障害有病者数の動向．日本では適応障害に罹患する人は春，夏，秋に増えて，冬に少ない傾向がある．うつ・適応障害の発症には，身体ストレスのほか，気候，環境，睡眠の変化など，生活上のストレスが影響していることが考えられる．
［健康保険組合連合会：平成25年度メンタル系疾患の動向に関するレポートより］

Reading 1

Vocabulary Study

以下の①〜⑩の語（句）の意味を a.〜j. から選びましょう．そのうえで実際に発音を練習してみましょう．

① amputate　　　　a. 大腿
② sarcoma　　　　 b. 仕切る
③ thigh　　　　　　c. 注視
④ stump　　　　　 d. 生命徴候
⑤ grieve　　　　　 e. 除去する
⑥ vital sign　　　　f. 切断する
⑦ gaze　　　　　　g. 断端，付け根
⑧ partition　　　　h. ひざ（座ったときの下腹部からひざ頭までの部分）
⑨ lap　　　　　　　i. 悲しむ
⑩ eliminate　　　　j. 肉腫

Kaori Akita is 17 years old. Five days ago, she had her left leg amputated above the knee to remove Ewing's sarcoma in the tibia. Her left thigh was treated with a stump plasty at ten centimeters above the knee joint. She grieved for the loss of her left leg and feared the recurrence of the cancer. She could not sleep well, and she ate less than half of the meals prepared for her.

Masao Ishii has worked as an occupational therapist for three years. He has been in charge of providing Kaori with rehabilitation services. Today he worked with her for the third time. He asked her how she was feeling, and she responded that she was not feeling well and that she did not feel like doing any exercises.

Masao checked her vital signs. Her temperature was 35.7 degrees, her blood pressure was 110 over 56, and her pulse was 70 beats per minute. He told her that her temperature, blood pressure, and pulse were all normal and suggested that she should do some exercises. She turned him down saying that she did not feel like standing up, and that she did not want anyone to see her. She felt that she was under the gaze of curious eyes.

He told her that the place she would undergo rehabilitation exercises was partitioned with curtains so that she would not be seen by others. He also told her that her lap would be covered with a rug in the wheelchair on the way to the rehabilitation room and the way back to her room. However, she did not respond to his suggestion. She just lamented over her misfortune saying that she could no longer walk, run or swim, and she felt a deep sense of loss.

Before the operation, Kaori understood that she had to have her left leg amputated. After the surgery, however, she felt miserable and came to dislike herself. She told Masao that having her leg amputated was much harder than she had expected and that she was scared that the cancer might recur. The doctor said that he had completely eliminated the cancer so she should focus on rehabilitation without any worries, but she was still very anxious.

Listening to Kaori, Masao understood that she was so depressed that she was not ready for rehabilitation exercises for daily living. He only gave her a passive range-of-motion exercise for her hip joints and decided to talk about her mental state with the doctor in charge.

Notes：Ewing's sarcoma ユーイング肉腫，tibia 脛骨，stump plasty 断端形成.

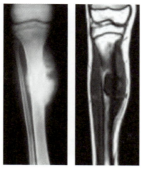

Figure. 脛骨に生じたユーイング肉腫

Reading Comprehension

本文の内容に一致するものには T（True），異なるものには F（False）を記入しましょう．

① Kaori had a surgery on her left foot five days ago.　（　）
② Kaori suffered from Ewing's sarcoma in the tibia.　（　）
③ Kaori has been afraid that she might have cancer again.　（　）
④ Masao has worked with Kaori for dozens of times.　（　）
⑤ Kaori did not want to do exercises, though Masao suggested that she should do them.　（　）
⑥ Masao tried to convince Kaori that she would get used to rehabilitation exercises.　（　）
⑦ Kaori expressed her worries to Masao.　（　）
⑧ Kaori focused on rehabilitation because the doctor encouraged her to do so.　（　）
⑨ Masao gave Kaori a passive range-of-motion exercise for her hip joints because she asked for it.　（　）
⑩ Masao decided to talk with the doctor to confirm that Kaori's operation was a success.　（　）

パーツと語源で覚える医学用語

●**sarcoma**　肉腫

　sarc(o)- は「肉（flesh）」の意のギリシャ語 *sarx* に由来する前部連結形．ギリシャ語系接尾辞 -oma は「腫・瘤（tumor）」の意．

Reading 2

Vocabulary Study

以下の①〜⑩の語（句）の意味を a.〜j. から選びましょう．そのうえで実際に発音を練習してみましょう．

① adjustment
② excessively
③ causative
④ pharmacotherapy
⑤ insomnia
⑥ manipulation
⑦ stressor
⑧ lower extremity prosthesis
⑨ verbalize
⑩ autonomous

a. 操作，扱い
b. 自律した
c. 適応
d. 言葉で表す
e. 義足
f. 不眠（症）
g. 原因となる
h. 薬物療法
i. ストレスを引き起こす要因
j. 過剰に

　Adjustment disorder is a condition that occurs when a person has great difficulty in coping with or adjusting to a particular condition or event and feels depressed and anxious. Patients are easily moved to tears and excessively worried about something. It is thought that adjustment disorder is almost the same as symptomatic depression or reactive depression that has a clear cause of stress.

　It is often the case that symptoms are reduced when the causative stress of adjustment disorder is alleviated. For example, when there is an issue to solve at work that engenders stress, this may give rise to feelings of anxiety and depression at the workplace. However, on the day off these feelings may disappear enough to enjoy hobbies.

　The situation or the event which creates stress is obvious; therefore, adjustment disorder is likely to be alleviated as the cause of stress disappears. However, symptoms may become chronic in cases where the cause of stress cannot be removed. Patients with irreversible impairment such as limb amputation are likely to feel a strong sense of loss and immense grief while undergoing rehabilitation. Cancer patients in the terminal stage who are conscious of their limited life span may emotionally and behaviorally deviate from the range of normality. It is not easy to change such conditions in patients. If they continuously feel depressed, enjoy no activities, have little appetite, and suffer from sleeplessness for a long time, they may be diagnosed with depression.

　Adjustment disorder can be treated with pharmacotherapy for insomnia, counseling, environmental manipulation, and coping skills training. Environmental manipulation includes elimination of the stressors of the patients. For example, Kaori worries about how she appears to others, so when she has training or uses a wheelchair, one way to avoid the stress is to cover her amputated leg with a lap rug. Another way is to use a temporary lower extremity prosthesis until she has her own made.

It is good to remove the cause of stress through environmental manipulation, but at times it is difficult. In such a case, behavioral training which fits the situation of patients with adjustment disorder should be used. For example, the patients can be given training to verbalize their problem or situation. In rehabilitation programs for patients with adjustment disorder, it is vital for the therapists to accept and understand the patients' feelings and help them become positive and autonomous.

> **Notes**：symptomatic depression 症候性うつ，reactive depression 反応性うつ．

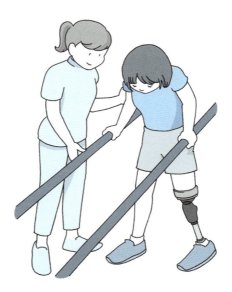

Comprehension Questions

以下の問いに英語で答えましょう．

① When does adjustment disorder happen?
② What symptoms do people with adjustment disorder have?
③ What kind of patients are likely to feel a strong sense of loss and immense grief while undergoing rehabilitation?
④ In what cases may individuals be diagnosed with depression?
⑤ What kind of medicine is mentioned in the reading?
⑥ What skill training is given as a treatment of adjustment disorder?
⑦ What should be removed from the environment for patients with adjustment disorder?
⑧ What environmental manipulation examples does the passage mention about Kaori's case?
⑨ What should be done if removing a cause of stress is difficult?
⑩ What should the therapists do for the rehabilitation of patients with adjustment disorder?

パーツと語源で覚える医学用語

● **irreversible** 不可逆的な

ir- は「不・無・非 (not)」の意のラテン語由来の接頭辞．ir-「不」+ reversible「逆にできる」=「不可逆的な」という構造．ir- は「不・無・非 (not)」の意の接頭辞 in- の異形である．この否定の接頭辞 in- は上の例のように，r の前にくるときに ir- となり（例：irregular），l の前では il- となり（例：illogical），b, m, p の前においては im- となる（例：impossible）．

● **pharmacotherapy** 薬物療法

pharmac(o)- は「薬 (drug)」の意のギリシャ語由来の前部連結形．therapy「治療・療法」と結び付いて薬物療法となる．cf. pharmacology「薬理学」，-logy「学問」

● **insomnia** 不眠(症)

簡単な英語で言えば sleeplessness のこと．in- は前述のとおり「不・無・非 (not)」の意のラテン語由来の接頭辞である．somnia の部分は「眠る (sleep)」の意のラテン語 somnus に由来し，語尾の -ia は名詞を作る接尾辞であり，しばしば病名にも現れる．

Dictation
録音を聴いて空欄を埋め，各英文を完成させましょう．
① The patient is easily (　　　　　　　　　　　　　　　　　　　　　) about something.
② Symptoms (　　　　　　　　　　　　　　　　　　　　) the cause of stress cannot be removed.
③ Adjustment disorder (　　　　　　　　　　　　　　　　　　　　　　　　　).

Composition
日本語の意味に合うように〔　〕内の語（句）を並べ替えましょう．必要に応じて「, 」を使用してください．

① その男性は，腕を失ったことを悲しみ，感染の恐れを抱いていた．
The man 〔 of, for, infection, the loss, his arm, feared, grieved, and 〕.

② 私の話を聞いて，作業療法士は私が落ち込んでいることを理解した．
〔 understood, to, occupational, listening, me, the, that, therapist 〕 I was depressed.

③ その患者の家族は，担当の医師と彼の薬について話したいと思った．
The patient's family 〔 charge, to, his medication, about, the doctor, wanted, talk, in, with 〕.

④ 障害を引き起こすストレスが軽減されると，症状は軽くなるだろう．
The symptom 〔 when, of, causative stress, reduced, the disorder, be, will, is, the 〕 alleviated.

⑤ 手足の切断のような不可逆的な障害のある患者は，強い喪失感を覚えるかもしれない．
Patients 〔 limb, as, may, loss, a strong sense, amputation, with, impairment, of, feel, irreversible, such 〕.

⑥ 深刻な問題に直面している人は，情緒面で正常範囲を逸脱するかもしれない．
Those 〔 emotionally deviate, face, who, may, serious, of, normality, a, from, the range, problem 〕.

⑦ 持続的に憂うつ気分が続けば，うつ病と診断されることがある．
If we continuously 〔 may, diagnosed, we, depression, depressed, be, feel, with 〕.

⑧ その女性は車いすに座るときは，脚をひざかけで覆う．
When 〔 in, covers, her wheelchair, a lap rug, she, her legs, sits, the woman, with 〕.

⑨ 適応障害の治療では，環境調整によりストレスの原因を取り除くことが大切である．
It is important 〔 stress, the, manipulation, by, to, environmental, remove, of, cause 〕 in the treatment of adjustment disorder.

⑩ 療法士は，患者の気持ちを受け入れ，彼らが自律するように手助けする必要がある．
Therapists 〔 help, to, feelings, autonomous, accept, and, them, become, need, the patients' 〕.

Medical Terms

第Ⅱ部のリスト（表 1 〜 3）を参考に，下記の語彙パーツを組み合わせて医学用語をつくり，日本語の意味も答えましょう．必要があれば同じパーツを何度使ってもかまいません．

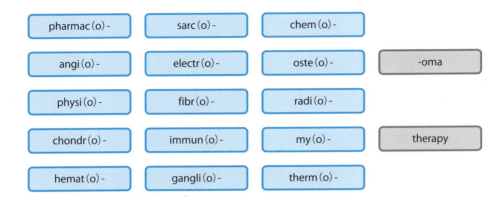

Let's try!

　In Reading 2, the author says, "In rehabilitation programs for patients with adjustment disorder, it is vital for the therapists to accept and understand the patients' feelings and help them become positive and autonomous."

　How can the therapists help the patients become positive and autonomous? Discuss the question in groups.

Unit 9

Parkinson's Disease（パーキンソン病）

　パーキンソン病という病名は 1817 年にこの病気を報告したイギリス人医師 James Parkinson（1755～1824）に由来します．パーキンソン病を発症すると，脳が出す運動の指令が筋に伝わりにくくなるため円滑な動作ができなくなってしまいます．主な初期症状としては，安静時の手足の震え（安静時振戦），固縮，無動，姿勢反射障害が挙げられますが，ほかにも便秘，排尿障害，立ちくらみ，といった自律神経症状や，うつ症状を伴う場合もあります．

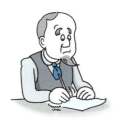
ふるえ（振戦）

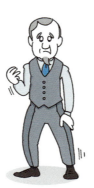
筋肉がこわばる（筋固縮）

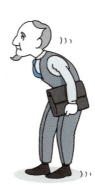
動作が遅くなる（無動）

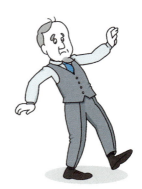
姿勢を保てなくなる（姿勢反射障害）

パーキンソン病の 4 大徴候

Reading 1

Vocabulary Study

以下の①～⑩の語（句）の意味を a.～j. から選びましょう．そのうえで実際に発音を練習してみましょう．

① conductor　　　　　a. 適切な
② be involved in　　　b. 指揮者
③ advise　　　　　　　c. ～を強める
④ facility　　　　　　　d. 例年の，毎年の
⑤ reunion　　　　　　e. 監督，管理
⑥ appropriate　　　　f. ～を優先させる
⑦ prioritize　　　　　 g. 同窓会，懇親会
⑧ strengthen　　　　 h. 施設，設備
⑨ supervision　　　　i. 助言する
⑩ annual　　　　　　 j.（活動などに）参加する，携わる

Tetsuo Kobayashi is a 70-year-old man, who loves music and has been playing an active role in a local orchestra as a conductor. He has been married to his wife, Chiaki, a violinist in the same orchestra, for 35 years. They met each other through music and got married, so being involved in the local orchestra has been more than just a favorite pastime.

However, Tetsuo started having trouble with mobility 10 years ago and became aware that he was more likely to fall. At age 65, he was diagnosed as having Parkinson's disease, and his attending doctor advised him to undergo rehabilitation twice a week. The disorder progressed gradually at the beginning, so he was able to continue his activities in the orchestra as a conductor in spite of his difficulty with walking and balance, as Chiaki always accompanied Tetsuo to provide assistance and make sure of his safety. But as the disorder progressed, the time came when Tetsuo had to use a wheelchair in his everyday life. One day, Tetsuo suddenly told Chiaki that he would quit the orchestra because he was not satisfied with his performance as a conductor. Chiaki knew that these were not his real feelings, she suggested to him that he continue his activities in the orchestra for a time. She also suggested that he go to a different hospital in a neighboring city that was known for its excellent rehabilitation programs and facilities. She had heard about this hospital from one of her classmates she had met at a high school class reunion. Tetsuo agreed with Chiaki, and they decided to visit the new hospital in an effort to find a way to minimize the effects of the disease so that Tetsuo could continue to do something in the orchestra.

Kyosuke Miura is a physical therapist who has been working for the hospital for four years. He talked with Tetsuo and Chiaki to better understand their lifestyle and set up an appropriate rehabilitation program. Kyosuke first thought of prioritizing rehabilitation aimed at strengthening Tetsuo's leg muscles to enable him to go to the toilet with the assistance of Chiaki at home. But Tetsuo asked him if more emphasis could be placed on rehabilitation that would enable him to use his arms more freely so that he would be able to continue to conduct the orchestra for some time. After listening to Chiaki and Tetsuo, Kyosuke decided to place more weight on rehabilitation for sitting balance and mobility of arms in Tetsuo's program. At the new hospital, Tetsuo underwent rehabilitation with a more positive attitude under the supervision of the young physical therapist who constantly encouraged him to improve his condition. In six months, Tetsuo appeared on the stage of the annual concert of their orchestra as the conductor in a wheelchair. Chiaki was pleased to see Tetsuo conducting the orchestra with a smile on his face.

Notes : real feelings 本心, place emphasis on〜/place weight on〜 〜に重きを置く，〜を重視する.

Reading Comprehension

本文の内容に一致するものにはT（True），異なるものにはF（False）を記入しましょう．

① Tetsuo and Chiaki have been involved in the same local orchestra for a long time.　（　　）

② It is 10 years since Chiaki had trouble with her mobility.　（　　）

③ Tetsuo was diagnosed as having Parkinson's disease five years ago.　（　　）

④ Chiaki was advised by the doctor to accompany Tetsuo at any time.　（　　）

⑤ Chiaki persuaded Tetsuo to continue his activities in the orchestra.　（　　）

⑥ Chiaki took Tetsuo to a different hospital so that he could slow down the progress of the disease because she wanted him to continue his activities in the orchestra.　（　　）

⑦ Kyosuke is an experienced physical therapist known for his outstanding skills.　（　　）

⑧ Tetsuo asked Kyosuke to strengthen his leg muscles so that he could go to the toilet without assistance.　（　　）

⑨ Tetsuo asked Kyosuke to enable him to conduct the orchestra for some time.　（　　）

⑩ The progress of Parkinson's disease prevented Tetsuo from appearing on the stage of the annual concert as a conductor.　（　　）

パーツと語源で覚える医学用語

● **disease** 病気，疾病，疾患
　dis- は「不〜，無〜，非〜」の意のラテン語由来の接頭辞．dis-（否定）＋ ease（安楽）＝「病気」．古フランス語 *desaise* より．文字どおり，病気になると「楽ではない」．

● **minimize** 最小にする
　minim(um)「最小の」＋ -ize ＝「〜の状態にする，〜化する」（ギリシャ語由来の接頭辞）．cf. maximize「最大にする」

● **supervision** 監督，管理
　ラテン語 *supervidere* に由来．super-（上に）＋ *videre*（見る）＝「監督」．

Reading 2

Vocabulary Study

以下の①~⑩の語（句）の意味を a.~j. から選びましょう．そのうえで実際に発音を練習してみましょう．

① motor system　　　　　a. 神経伝達物質
② neurotransmitter　　　 b.（観察によって）認める，気づく
③ reduction　　　　　　　c. 前かがみの
④ tremor　　　　　　　　 d. 呼吸器の
⑤ rigidity　　　　　　　　e. 振戦，震え
⑥ involuntary　　　　　　f. 運動系
⑦ observe　　　　　　　 g. 不随意の，意思によらない
⑧ stooped　　　　　　　 h. 減少
⑨ droop　　　　　　　　 i. 固縮
⑩ respiratory　　　　　　j. 垂れる，下げる

　Parkinson's disease is a progressive disorder of the central nervous system primarily affecting the motor system. It is most common among men in the 50-60 age group, but it can also attack women and young people. It is estimated that approximately one out of every 1,000 Japanese people develops the disorder.

　Parkinson's disease affects nerve cells in the brain responsible for planning and controlling body movement. It has been confirmed among patients with Parkinson's disease that there is a reduction in the number of nerve cells, called neurons, in an area of the brain called the substantia nigra. The neurons produce dopamine, which functions as a neurotransmitter that sends messages to the area of the brain that controls movement and coordination. Therefore, the reduction in the number of the dopamine-producing nerve cells can generate problems in controlling movement.

　The most common symptoms of the disorder are resting tremor, rigidity, akinesia or bradykinesia, and postural instability. Tremor is the repetitive, involuntary shaking of body parts, such as the hands and arms. Resting tremors occur while sitting and being relaxed. Rigidity means stiff and inflexible muscles caused by uncontrolled tensing of muscles, which prevents moving about freely. Akinesia is defined as a loss of controllable motion, and bradykinesia refers to slowness of movement. These symptoms are observed when patients with Parkinson's try to start walking or roll over in bed. Postural instability refers to the state in which it is difficult to keep the body in a stable position. This symptom is due to the loss of postural reflexes, and can cause the patients to have a stooped posture in which the head is bowed and the shoulders are drooped. Postural instability often affects a patient's walking, and his steps may become shorter and shorter as if he were hurrying forward to keep balance. Other symptoms include depression, urinary urgency and frequency, insomnia, a serious-looking face called masking, and dysphagia. But symptoms of Parkinson's vary from person to person, as does the rate of progression. The progression of the disease is commonly classified into five stages using the Hoehn and Yahr scale corresponding to the severity of movement symptoms and to the degree the disease affects a person's everyday activities.

There is currently no cure for Parkinson's disease, but treatments including medications and proper rehabilitation programs can help control the symptoms and maintain the patient's quality of life. A physical therapist will develop a program to help the patient stay as independent as possible and prescribe exercises and techniques to deal with the condition, focusing on improving balance, walking and overall functional ability. As the disease will finally affect the patient's swallowing and breathing functions, exercises focusing on swallowing and breathing will be started prior to the onset of dysphagia and respiratory problems.

> **Notes**：substantia nigra 黒質（ドーパミンをつくる中脳にある神経細胞），resting tremor 安静時振戦，akinesia 無動，失動，bradykinesia 動作緩慢，postural instability 姿勢反射障害（姿勢の不安定），loss of postural reflexes 姿勢反射の喪失，urinary urgency and frequency 尿意逼迫と頻尿，masking 仮面様顔貌，dysphagia 嚥下障害，the Hoehn and Yahr scale ホーエン・ヤールの重症度分類．

Comprehension Questions

以下の問いに英語で答えましょう．

① In what age group is Parkinson's disease most common?
② What is the incidence of Parkinson's disease among Japanese people?
③ In what area of the brain of a patient with Parkinson's disease can a reduction in the number of neurons be found?
④ What are the major symptoms of Parkinson's disease?
⑤ What is akinesia?
⑥ What is bradykinesia?
⑦ What causes postural instability in patients with Parkinson's disease?
⑧ What is a serious looking face of a patient with Parkinson's disease called?
⑨ What is the medical term for the difficulty in swallowing?
⑩ How can patients with Parkinson's disease be treated?

パーツと語源で覚える医学用語

- **neurotransmitter** 神経伝達物質
  neur(o)- は「神経 (nerve), 神経系 (the nervous system)」の意のギリシャ語由来の前部連結形. neuro- ＋ transmitter「伝達物質」＝「神経伝達物質」.

- **akinesia** 無動, 失動（随意運動能力の喪失や障害）
  a-「無 (without)」については Unit 6 と Unit 10 を参照. -kinesia は「運動 (movement)」の意のギリシャ語由来の後部連結形. a-「無」＋ -kinesia「運動」＝「無動」.

- **bradykinesia** 動作緩慢
  brady- は「遅い (slow)」の意のギリシャ語由来の前部連結形. brady-「遅い」＋ -kinesia「運動」＝「動作緩慢」.

- **insomnia** 不眠
  Unit 8 を参照.

- **dysphagia** 嚥下障害
  -phagia「食べること (eating)」はギリシャ語由来の後部連結形. dys-「悪化」＋ -phagia「食べること」＝「嚥下障害」. dys-「悪化 (bad)」については Unit 3 を参照.

Dictation

録音を聴いて空欄を埋め，各英文を完成させましょう．

① Chiaki always (　　　　　　　　　　　　　　　　) his safety.

② He decided to (　　　　　　　　　　　　　　　　) for sitting balance.

③ It (　　　　　　　　　　　　　　　　) Parkinson's disease that there is a reduction in the number of nerve cells.

Composition

日本語の意味に合うように〔　〕内の語（句）を並べ替えましょう．必要に応じて「,」を使用してください．

① その医者は認知症を予防しようとして，血糖値と認知症の関係を調べた．

The doctor examined the link 〔 between, levels, an, effort, and, to, dementia, in, blood sugar, prevent 〕 the disease.

② その医者は松葉杖を使うように提案したが，私は嫌だった．

The 〔 I, use, crutches, suggested, doctor, that 〕, but I didn't want to do so.

③ このプログラムは自然との交流を強調しています．

This 〔 with, program, on, interaction, nature, places, emphasis 〕.

④ 医師は患者が病気に対する感情や心配を述べるように促すために制約のない質問をした．

The doctor asked the patient 〔 questions, her, to, describe, and concerns, to, encourage, her feelings, open-ended 〕 about her illness.

⑤ 国内で300万人がこの病気にかかっていると推定されている．

It 〔 from, people nationwide, 3 million, estimated, that, suffer, is 〕 this disease.

⑥ その病院は患者の減少から昨年の春に小児科を廃止した．

The hospital closed 〔 to, a decrease, its, department, last spring, the, number, due, pediatrics, in 〕 of patients.

⑦ この病気の初期症状は寒気，熱，そして喉の痛みである．

The 〔 disease, of, this, fever, include, chills, symptoms, initial 〕, and sore throat.

⑧ 骨粗鬆症は骨量減少と骨の劣化によって引き起こされる病気である．

Osteoporosis 〔 bone, a, disease, by, low, caused, is, bone mass, and 〕 deterioration.

⑨ 睡眠障害は3つの主要なカテゴリーに分類される．

Sleep 〔 into, major, three, are, classified, categories, disorders 〕.

⑩ われわれの研究はその伝染病の蔓延防止に焦点を合わせている．

Our 〔 the contagious, the spread, of, on, preventing, research, focuses 〕 disease.

Medical Terms

第Ⅱ部のリスト（表1〜3）を参考に，空欄（1）〜（10）の接辞，連結形，語の意味を調べたうえで，それらを使って，日本語の意味に合うように空欄〔11〕〜〔20〕を埋めましょう。

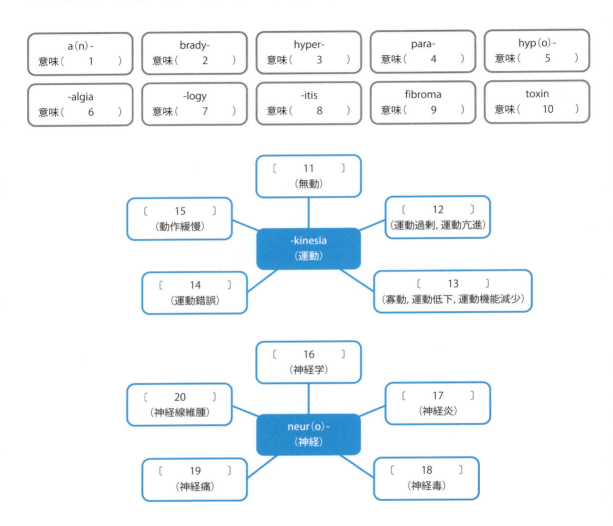

Let's try!

　As is mentioned in the passage, the Hoehn and Yahr scale is widely used to describe the symptoms in the progression of Parkinson's disease. Search the Web for more detailed information on the five stages of the disease. Then make a pair and share your information with your partner.

Unit 10
Cerebrovascular Disease（脳血管障害）

　脳血管障害には，血管の閉塞や狭窄により血流が悪くなって起こる虚血性脳血管障害と，血管が破れて生じる出血性脳血管障害があります．障害のある人には，リハビリテーションとして，理学療法，作業療法，言語聴覚療法などが処方されます．脳血管疾患を予防するためには，高血圧にならないように塩分の多いものや脂肪の多いものを控えてバランスのよい食事をとること，過度な飲酒を避けること，禁煙や運動を心がけることなど，生活習慣を改善していくことが重要になります．

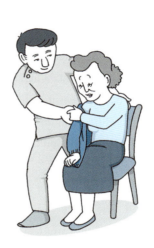

右上下肢に運動麻痺を呈した脳血管障害患者の日常生活動作練習の様子

Reading 1

Vocabulary Study

以下の①～⑩の語（句）の意味を a.～j. から選びましょう．そのうえで実際に発音を練習してみましょう．

① groan　　　　　　　　a. 不可欠な，必須の
② cerebral　　　　　　　b.（脳）神経外科（学）
③ infarction　　　　　　c. 入院
④ artery　　　　　　　　d. うなる
⑤ hemisphere　　　　　　e. 肺の
⑥ neurosurgery　　　　　f. 口頭で
⑦ pulmonary　　　　　　g. 動脈
⑧ hospitalization　　　　h. 半球
⑨ orally　　　　　　　　i. 梗塞
⑩ integral　　　　　　　j. 脳の，大脳の

Unit 10 Cerebrovascular Disease（脳血管障害）

Shinya Miyamoto is 65 years old. He has suffered from high blood pressure and diabetes since he was about 50 years old. One day, when he woke up in the morning, he could not move his right hand well. He tried to stand up, but his right knee was not strong enough to support him, which caused him to fall down on the futon. When his wife heard him falling, she asked him if he was all right, but he only groaned. She immediately called an ambulance, and it took him to a hospital. He was diagnosed with cerebral infarction.

Shinya had infarction of his left middle cerebral artery, and he was not able to talk due to the involvement of Broca's area located in the left hemisphere of the brain, which plays a vital role in speech production. In addition, he was unable to manipulate his right limbs. He attempted to move his right arm, but he could not. He felt that his right leg was very heavy like a log. He was worried that his right limbs could not move, and he was also anxious that he could not talk though he could come up with some words.

After having received medical treatment in the department of neurosurgery at the hospital, Shinya was admitted to the recovery rehabilitation unit. When he was in a supine position on the bed, his doctor came. She told him to raise his right hand higher than his head. He was able to slightly flex his right elbow and move his fingers one centimeter. She told him to close his mouth and puff his cheeks up, but he could not close the right side of his mouth. Without pulmonary aspiration he was able to drink water from a small feeding cup.

The doctor prescribed exercise therapy for his right upper and lower limbs, ADL training, and speech therapy for his rehabilitation. She instructed him to start physical therapy, occupational therapy, and speech therapy three days after his hospitalization. She told the occupational therapist in charge that Shinya should practice intensively using his right hand and also practice writing with his left hand, because he might have to communicate in writing were he to become unable to orally communicate, and it would be hard for him to write with his right hand as well as he did before. Therefore, to practice using his left hand effectively would be an integral part of his rehabilitation.

Notes：**left middle cerebral artery** 左中大脳動脈，**Broca's area** ブローカ野，**supine position** 背臥位，**pulmonary aspiration** 誤嚥．

Reading Comprehension

本文の内容に一致するものにはT（True），異なるものにはF（False）を記入しましょう．

① Shinya has had high blood pressure and diabetes for about 50 years.　（　　）
② Shinya fell down because his right knee was not strong enough to support him.　（　　）
③ Shinya was unable to answer his wife's question when he fell down.　（　　）
④ Shinya's wife drove him to the hospital.　（　　）
⑤ The doctor told Shinya that he had had a heart attack.　（　　）
⑥ Shinya was hospitalized after he received medical treatment.　（　　）
⑦ Shinya practiced drinking water in the rehabilitation program.　（　　）
⑧ Shinya was instructed to start exercise therapy for his left arm and leg.　（　　）
⑨ The doctor instructed Shinya to start physical therapy, occupational therapy, and speech therapy.　（　　）
⑩ The doctor said that Shinya should alternately use his right hand and left hand.　（　　）

パーツと語源で覚える医学用語

● **neurosurgery**　（脳）神経外科(学)

　neur(o)- は「神経（nerve），神経系（nervous system）」の意（Unit 9 の neurotransmitter を参照）．neuro- + surgery「外科」=「(脳) 神経外科」．

● **pulmonary**　肺の

　pulmon(o)- は「肺（lung）」の意のラテン語由来の前部連結形．ラテン語由来の接尾辞 -ary は「～の，～に関する」の意の形容詞語尾．

Reading 2

Vocabulary Study

以下の①〜⑩の語（句）の意味を a.〜j. から選びましょう．そのうえで実際に発音を練習してみましょう．

① mortality rate　　　　a. 閉塞
② stroke　　　　　　　　b. 頭蓋骨
③ ischemic　　　　　　　c. 頭蓋の，頭部の
④ obstruction　　　　　 d. 予後
⑤ intracerebral　　　　　e. 出血
⑥ hemorrhage　　　　　 f. 脳内の
⑦ skull　　　　　　　　　g. 脳卒中
⑧ prognosis　　　　　　 h. 死亡率
⑨ hemiplegia　　　　　　i. 虚血性の
⑩ cranial　　　　　　　　j. 片麻痺

　In Japan, cerebrovascular disease is the fourth most common cause of death preceded by cancer, heart failure, and pulmonary disease. Even though the mortality rate for cerebrovascular disease is falling due to medical development, the disease is likely to cause patients to become bedridden because of motor impairment. The number of patients suffering from a stroke remains high in this society which has aged and seen an increase in lifestyle-related diseases. Therefore, the treatment and prevention of stroke has become an important issue.

　One type of cerebrovascular disease is ischemic cerebrovascular disease caused by vascular obstruction and angiostenosis leading to poor blood flow. The other kind is hemorrhagic cerebrovascular disease resulting from the rupture of blood vessels. Ischemic cerebrovascular disease comprises cerebral infarction and transient ischemic attack. Hemorrhagic cerebrovascular disease has two types of hemorrhage: intracerebral hemorrhage and subarachnoid hemorrhage. Intracerebral hemorrhage is bleeding within the brain tissue, while subarachnoid hemorrhage is bleeding into the space surrounding the brain. In subarachnoid hemorrhage, blood leaks from blood vessels to the surface of the brain, and the bleeding occurs in the arteries that run underneath a membrane called the arachnoid, which is located just below the surface of the skull. Treatment includes stopping the bleeding and relieving the pressure on the brain. There also exist treatments relevant to each disease or condition. Appropriate diagnosis and immediate treatment should have a positive influence on the prognosis of the patients.

　Physical disability due to a stroke includes motility disturbance such as hemiplegia and ataxia. Right and left motor nerve tracts that go to the limbs from the brain cross in the brainstem; therefore, if one of the cerebral hemispheres is damaged, the contralateral limbs suffer from motor impairment. Sensory disturbance such as pain also occurs.

Furthermore, a stroke can result in brain dysfunction such as disturbance of consciousness, dementia, aphasia, agnosia, and apraxia. The symptoms of a stroke vary and include cranial nerve disorders such as ocular motility disorder, dysarthria and dysphagia.

Stroke rehabilitation is divided into the acute phase, the convalescent phase, and the maintenance phase. In the acute phase, patients engage in motor learning, and their goal is to achieve early independence for self-care right from the onset. In the convalescence phase, they aim for prompt recovery of physical functions. Rehabilitation in the maintenance phase is administered for the upkeep of the acquired functions as long as possible.

> **Notes**: angiostenosis 血管狭窄, hemorrhagic 出血性, subarachnoid hemorrhage くも膜下出血, ataxia 運動失調（症）, aphasia 失語（症）, agnosia 失認（症）, apraxia 失行（症）, ocular motility disorder 眼球運動障害, dysarthria 構音障害, convalescent phase 回復期.

Comprehension Questions

以下の問いに英語で答えましょう．

① What are the four major causes of death in Japan?
② Why is the mortality rate for cerebrovascular disease going down?
③ What increase do we see in the modern aged society?
④ What do vascular obstruction and angiostenosis cause?
⑤ What causes hemorrhagic cerebrovascular disease?
⑥ Where do right and left motor nerve tracts that go to the limbs from the brain cross?
⑦ What does the rehabilitation for strokes comprise?
⑧ What do patients aim at in the acute phase?
⑨ What is the goal of the convalescence phase?
⑩ In what phase do patients try to keep up the acquired functions?

パーツと語源で覚える医学用語

- **cerebrovascular** 脳血管の
  Unit 5 を参照.

- **angiostenosis** 血管狭窄（症）
  angi(o)- は「血管（blood vessel）」の意のギリシャ語由来の前部連結形. angio- + stenosis「狭窄（症）」=「血管狭窄（症）」. stenosis「狭窄（症）」は Unit 5 を参照.

- **hemorrhage/haemorrhage** （多量の）出血
  hem(o)-/haem(o)- は「血液（blood）」の意のギリシャ語由来の前部連結形. -rrhage は「異常排出・流出過多（excessive and abnormal flow）」の意のギリシャ語由来の後部連結形.

- **intracerebral** 脳内の
  ラテン語由来の接頭辞 intra-「内の（within/inside）」+ cerebral「脳の（brain）」=「脳内の」. cerebr(o)-「脳（brain）」は Unit 5 の cerebrovascular を参照.

- **subarachnoid** くも膜下の
  sub- は「下の（under）」の意のラテン語由来の接頭辞. sub- + arachnoid「くも膜・くも膜の」=「くも膜下の」. また，arachn(o)- は「くも（spider），くも膜」の意のギリシャ語由来の前部連結形. -oid は「〜に似た（like）」の意のギリシャ語由来の接尾辞.

- **prognosis** 予後
  Unit 3 を参照.

- **hemiplegia** 片麻痺
  ギリシャ語由来の接頭辞 hemi-「半分」+ -plegia「麻痺」=「半側麻痺」. 後部連結形 -plegia については Unit 7 の解説および練習問題 Medical Terms を参照.

- **dysfunction** 機能障害
  Unit 3 を参照.

- **ataxia** 運動失調（症），**aphasia** 失語（症），**agnosia** 失認（症），**apraxia** 失行（症）
  a-/an- は「不・無・非（not/without）」の意のギリシャ語由来の接頭辞. ギリシャ語由来の後部連結形 -taxia「秩序（order）」, -phasia「言語障害（speech disorder）」, -gnosia「認識（recognition）」, -praxia「動作（action）」と結び付いて，それぞれ「運動失調」「失語」「失認」「失行」となる.

- **contralateral** （体の）反対側の
  contra- は「反対・逆（against/opposite）」の意のラテン語由来の接頭辞. contra- + lateral「外側の，側方の」=「（体の）反対側の」.

- **dysarthria** 構音障害
  dys-「困難な（difficult）」+ ギリシャ語 arthron「継ぎ目」=「構音障害」.

- **dysphagia** 嚥下障害
  dys- (difficult) + -phagia (eating) =「嚥下障害」. Unit 9 を参照.

Dictation

録音を聴いて空欄を埋め，各英文を完成させましょう．

① The doctor （   ） his right upper and lower limbs.

② To practice using your left hand effectively would be （   ）.

③ Cerebrovascular disease is likely to cause patients to （   ）.

Composition

日本語の意味に合うように〔 〕内の語（句）を並べ替えましょう．必要に応じて「,」を使用してください．

① 左脳には，発語において重要な役割を果たすブローカ野がある．

Located in the left hemisphere of the brain is Broca's area, 〔 an, production, plays, in, role, which, important, speech 〕.

② 祖父は治療を受けた後，回復期のリハビリテーション病棟へ入院した．

After having received medical treatment, my grandfather 〔 the, was, rehabilitation unit, to, admitted, recovery 〕.

③ 医師は，患者が右手を使う練習をする必要があると，作業療法士に伝えた．

The doctor told〔 the, the, occupational, practice, that, patient, should, his right hand, therapist, using 〕.

④ 脳内出血は，脳細胞内の出血であり，一方くも膜下出血は，脳を包囲するスペースへの出血である．

Intracerebral hemorrhage is bleeding within the brain tissue, 〔 is, the space, bleeding, the brain, surrounding, subarachnoid hemorrhage, while, into 〕.

⑤ くも膜と呼ばれる膜は，頭蓋骨の表面のすぐ下に位置している．

A membrane called the arachnoid 〔 below, just, the, the, located, of, is, skull, surface 〕.

⑥ 治療には，出血を止めることと脳圧を下げることが含まれる．

Treatment includes stopping 〔 bleeding, on, pressure, brain, relieving, and, the, the, the 〕.

⑦ それぞれの疾患には適した治療法がある．

There 〔 each, relevant, treatments, to, disease, exist 〕.

⑧ 適切な診断と早急な治療が患者の予後によい影響を与えるはずである．

Appropriate diagnosis and immediate treatment 〔 the, the, prognosis, a positive, on, of, have, should, influence, patients 〕.

⑨ 脳半球の一方が損傷すると，その反対側の手足が運動障害をこうむる．

If one of the cerebral hemispheres is damaged, 〔 impairment, motor, from, limbs, the contralateral, suffer 〕.

⑩ 患者たちは，急性期において発症直後から運動療法に取り組んでいる．

The patients 〔 the, the, in, in, exercise, phase, motor, right, from, acute, onset, engage 〕.

Medical Terms

第Ⅱ部のリスト（表1～3）を参考に，空欄（1）～（8）の後部連結形の意味を調べたうえで，例にならって空欄〔9〕～〔16〕を埋めましょう．

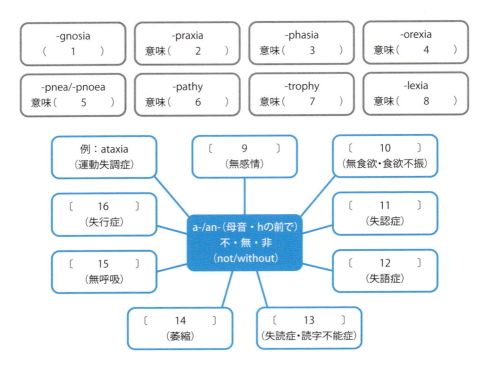

Let's try!

If a patient needed to practice writing with his left hand but he did not want to, what would you do as a therapist? Discuss the question in groups.

Unit 11

Dementia（認知症）

　高齢化の進展に伴い，さらに認知症の人が増えていくことが予測され，その対応は重要な課題のひとつとなっています．厚生労働省は，関係省庁と共同で，認知症施策推進総合戦略を策定しました．このなかには，認知症の容態に応じた適時・適切な医療・介護などの提供，認知症の予防法・診断法・治療法・リハビリテーションモデル・介護モデルなどの研究開発およびその成果の普及の推進に加えて，認知症の人の介護者への支援，認知症への理解を深めるための啓発の推進なども含まれています．

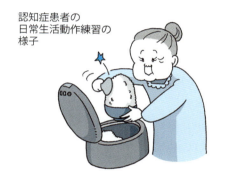

認知症患者の日常生活動作練習の様子

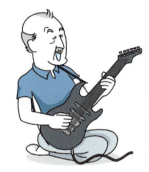

認知症患者は記憶力や思考力の低下が認められる一方，体得した技能は保存されやすい．

Reading 1

Vocabulary Study

以下の①～⑩の語（句）の意味を a.～j. から選びましょう．そのうえで実際に発音を練習してみましょう．

① irritable　　　　　　　　　　a. 安心な
② deteriorate　　　　　　　　　b. 拡大，膨張
③ despite　　　　　　　　　　　c. 不正確に
④ the neurology department　　 d. 不安な
⑤ inaccurately　　　　　　　　 e. 怒りっぽい
⑥ expansion　　　　　　　　　　f. 休息
⑦ mild cognitive impairment　　g. 神経内科
⑧ uneasy　　　　　　　　　　　 h. 悪化する
⑨ respite　　　　　　　　　　　i. ～にもかかわらず
⑩ secure　　　　　　　　　　　 j. 軽度認知障害

Yoshi Takagi is a 75-year-old woman. She lives with her eldest son and his wife in Yamanashi. She handed over her dairy farming business to them ten years ago and helped them with the work. She enjoyed taking a walk in and around the cow-house checking the cows and the grass fields every morning.

About a year ago, however, Yoshi became irritable and started to complain about the dairy farming and the meals that her family prepared. The relationship between Yoshi and her family deteriorated.

She often forgot that she had already eaten. After breakfast she asked her daughter-in-law whether breakfast was ready or not. Moreover, she thought that they did not have sufficient feed for the cows, and despite the fact that they had enough, she ordered it on her own without consulting anyone. She also went out for walks alone in the middle of the night. Her family wondered if she was showing signs of dementia and took her to the neurology department of the nearby hospital. She got upset on her arrival, but she gradually calmed down and agreed to have a medical examination.

The doctor asked her what day it was, but she answered the question inaccurately. He also asked her to subtract 7 from 93, and her answer was wrong. She was able to say the names of vegetables and fruits in a picture but could not remember the name of the governor who had recently taken office.

The doctor did not find apparent cerebral infarction or hemorrhage from her brain images but suspected hydrocephalus due to expansion of her cerebral ventricle and cerebral sulcus. She was diagnosed with mild cognitive impairment caused by hydrocephalus.

Yoshi was treated by the hospital staff that included Akio Sasaki, an occupational therapist. When he talked to her about the weather, she did not reply to his question but asked if her family had paid for the cows' feed. He also asked her about activities that she enjoyed. She did not answer the question but asked where her daughter-in-law was. She did not respond to his questions and repeatedly asked about the cows' feed and her daughter-in-law. She looked around the therapy room and seemed to feel uneasy.

She was told to regularly come to the hospital for intensive rehabilitation training for three months, which allowed her family a respite from her care. It is said that rehabilitation training for people with dementia is not only for them but also for their families. Akio planned to make the hospital environment comfortable for Yoshi so that she would feel secure and have a better cognitive understanding of her surroundings.

Notes：**hydrocephalus** 水頭症，**cerebral ventricle** 脳室，**cerebral sulcus** 脳溝．

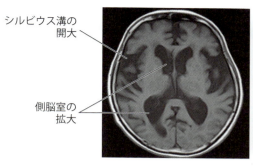
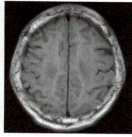

シルビウス溝の開大
側脳室の拡大

Figure. ヨシさんの脳画像
脳室と脳溝が拡大し，脳萎縮が著明（左）．その一方，高位の脳断面（右）では脳溝が不鮮明で，単なる脳萎縮ではなく水頭症が疑われる．

Reading Comprehension

本文の内容に一致するものにはT（True），異なるものにはF（False）を記入しましょう．

① Yoshi has been in the dairy farming business for ten years.　(　)
② Yoshi walked around the cow-shed every day.　(　)
③ The relationship between Yoshi and her family has always been good.　(　)
④ Yoshi often forgot to eat.　(　)
⑤ As Yoshi did not have sufficient feed for the cows, she ordered it.　(　)
⑥ Yoshi was taken to the hospital near her house by her family.　(　)
⑦ The doctor who examined Yoshi said that she had mild cognitive impairment caused by hydrocephalus.　(　)
⑧ Yoshi did not communicate well with Akio Sasaki, her occupational therapist.　(　)
⑨ Yoshi was told to come to the hospital for three months, and her family was asked to come with her.　(　)
⑩ Akio tried to help Yoshi respond appropriately to the questions.　(　)

パーツと語源で覚える医学用語

- **dementia** 認知症
  Unit 1 を参照．

- **neurology** 神経学
  -(o)logy は「学問（study of）」の意のギリシャ語由来の前部連結形．neur(o)- は「神経（nerve）神経系（the nervous system）」の意．（Unit 9 の neurotransmitter，Unit 10 の neurosurgery を参照．

- **hemorrhage** （多量の）出血
  Unit 10 を参照．

- **hydrocephalus** 水頭症
  hydr(o)- は「水（water）」の意のギリシャ語由来の前部連結形．-cephalus は「頭部異常（abnormal condition of the head）」の意のギリシャ語由来の後部連結形．

Reading 2

Vocabulary Study

以下の①～⑩の語（句）の意味を a.～j. から選びましょう．そのうえで実際に発音を練習してみましょう．

① decline　　　　　a. 複数の
② multiple　　　　 b. 言語の
③ competence　　 c. 介入
④ linguistic　　　 d. 示す，見せる
⑤ prevalence　　　e. 残存の
⑥ obvious　　　　 f. 刺激
⑦ reveal　　　　　 g. 有病率
⑧ residual　　　　 h. 低下
⑨ intervention　　 i. 能力
⑩ stimulus　　　　 j. 明らかな

　Dementia is a general term that describes a difficult situation in life caused by cognitive impairment. It is not a specific disease but a range of symptoms with a decline in memory and thinking abilities which disturb activities of daily living. When a person suffers greatly from multiple symptoms such as memory loss and decline of communicative competence, linguistic competence, concentration, logical thinking, judgment, and visual cognition, he or she may be diagnosed as having dementia.

　Alzheimer's disease is the most common type of dementia, and it accounts for more than 60 percent of cases. Vascular dementia, which is the second most common dementia type, is often caused by a stroke.

　People show a higher prevalence of dementia as they get older. However, young people may suffer from Alzheimer's disease and cerebrovascular diseases which may eventuate in dementia. Dementia diagnosed under the age of 65 is commonly described as younger or early onset dementia. Patients with younger or early onset dementia are at the working age but find it difficult to work or do housework due to the decline in memory and judgment, so they suffer from harsh living circumstances.

　Individuals who can manage their daily life independently in spite of an obvious memory decline may be diagnosed with mild cognitive impairment（MCI）. Those with MCI are likely to forget that they had a meal or what they ate, but they can eat on their own. Those with dementia, on the other hand, may forget that they are having a meal while eating. They are likely to forget what they ate or the fact that they had a meal, and the relationships with other people may deteriorate by their blaming them or revealing anger to them. Most individuals in the advanced stage of dementia do not admit that they have dementia, and it is hard to have them recognize what is happening to them.

　Rehabilitation for persons with dementia generally aims at improving cognitive functions and quality of life (QOL); however, in spite of careful rehabilitation, prominent improvements of the condition sometimes cannot be expected. In these cases, the aim of rehabilitation is to motivate patients and enhance their learning ability by helping them have a good time with others and activate their brain with positive and comfortable stimuli. These actions can help them become active and reinforce their residual ability.

Rehabilitation should be based on the following principles:

1. To make intervention for the patient a comfortable stimulus for him or her
2. To encourage communication between the patient and other people
3. To help the patient have a role to play and lead a life worth living
4. To repeatedly support favorable behavior

Note: vascular dementia 脳血管性認知症.

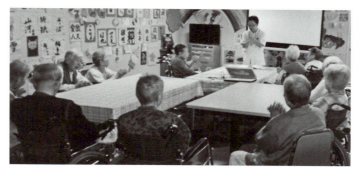

認知症の人に対するリハビリテーションの様子

Comprehension Questions

以下の問いに英語で答えましょう．

① What does a decline in memory and thinking abilities interfere with?
② What symptoms may persons with dementia suffer from?
③ What is the most common type of dementia?
④ What can lead to vascular dementia?
⑤ What is dementia diagnosed under the age of 65 commonly called?
⑥ What are individuals with mild cognitive impairment capable of?
⑦ How may persons with dementia harm the relationships with other people?
⑧ What kind of patients are unlikely to believe that they have dementia?
⑨ What is the general aim of the rehabilitation for those with dementia?
⑩ What needs to be supported over and over again in dementia rehabilitation?

パーツと語源で覚える医学用語

● **linguistic** 言語の
　lingu(o)- は「言語（language），舌（tongue）」の意のラテン語由来の前部連結形．-istic は形容詞をつくるギリシャ語由来の接尾辞．

● **cerebrovascular** 脳血管の
　Unit 5 を参照．

● **circumstance** 環境，周囲の事情，境遇
　circum-「周囲の（around）」はラテン語 circum（round）に由来する接頭辞．circumstance はラテン語 circumstare「取り囲む」に由来．circum- + stare「立つ（stand）」の構造．

● **diagnose** 診断する
　Unit 3 を参照．

Dictation
録音を聴いて空欄を埋め，各英文を完成させましょう．
① Dementia is a general term that (　　　　　　　　　　　　　　　　　) in life caused by cognitive impairment.
② Vascular dementia, which is the second most common dementia type, (　　　　　　　　　　　　　　　　　).
③ Most individuals in (　　　　　　　　　　　　　　　　　) do not admit that they have dementia.

Composition
日本語の意味に合うように〔　〕内の語（句）を並べ替えましょう．必要に応じて「,」を使用してください．
① その女性は，軽度認知障害と診断されて驚いた．
The woman〔 she, cognitive, mild, diagnosed, was, that, was, impairment, with, surprised 〕.
② その男性は，リハビリテーションのために病院に来たが，それで彼の家族は休息時間をとることになった．
The man〔 to, for, came, which, a respite, allowed, the hospital, rehabilitation training, his family 〕.
③ デイケアは，サービス利用者のためだけではなく，家族のためでもあると言われている．
It〔 but, that, also, is, is, day care, only, families, said, their, the service users, not, for, for 〕.
④ 高齢者のなかには，日常生活活動を妨げる記憶力の低下を示す人がいる．
Some elderly people〔 living, which, daily, disturbs, in, show, of, memory, activities, a decline 〕.
⑤ 患者は高齢になるにつれて，慢性疾患の有病率が高くなる．
Patients have〔 get, as, diseases, of, chronic, prevalence, they, older, higher, a 〕.
⑥ 65歳未満で診断された認知症は，通常若年性認知症と呼ばれる．
Dementia〔 under, dementia, or early, 65, usually, as, diagnosed, described, is, of, onset, the age, younger 〕.
⑦ その患者は，記憶力や判断力の低下により，仕事をすることが困難であるとわかっている．
The patient〔 it, to, to, in, judgment, due, work, finds, difficult, memory and, a decline 〕.
⑧ 軽度認知障害の人は，自分で食事ができる．
Those〔 impairment, their, mild, own, can, with, on, cognitive, eat 〕.
⑨ 注意深いリハビリテーションにもかかわらず，状況の著しい改善は，時に期待できない．
〔 improvements, careful, in, prominent, spite, rehabilitation, the condition, of, of 〕sometimes cannot be expected.
⑩ 患者への介入は，彼らにとって快刺激とするべきである．
We should〔 stimulus, for, for, a comfortable, make, them, patients, intervention 〕.

Medical Terms

第Ⅱ部のリスト（表1〜3）を参考に，空欄（1）〜（11）の前部連結形の意味を調べたうえで，例にならって空欄〔12〕〜〔21〕を埋めましょう．

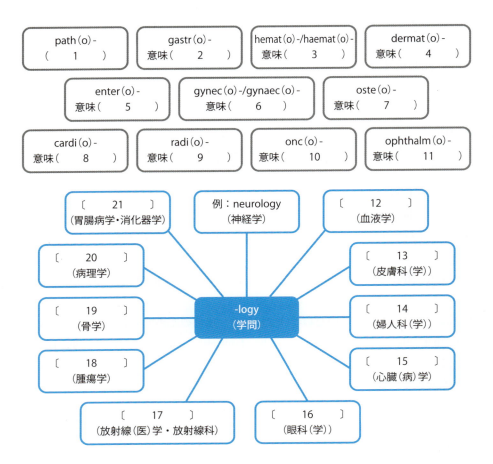

Let's try!

What do you think can help prevent dementia? Discuss the question in groups.

Unit 12

Diabetes Mellitus（糖尿病）

　糖尿病は体が必要とするインスリンを十分に産生しないため，食後に血糖値が異常に高くなる病気です．1型糖尿病では，膵臓のインスリン産生細胞が破壊されたため，インスリンをほとんど，またはまったくつくれなくなります．2型糖尿病では，膵臓はインスリンをつくり続けていますが，インスリン分泌が少なくなったり，体がインスリンの抵抗性を示し，あまりインスリンに反応しなくなったりします．糖尿病の治療では，食事療法，運動療法，そして多くの場合，薬物療法が行われます．血糖値をできる限り正常範囲に維持するようにコントロールしていれば，合併症は起こりにくくなります．

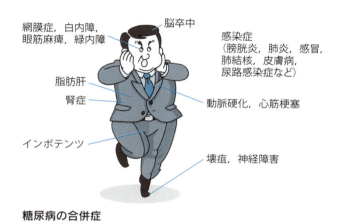

糖尿病の合併症

Reading 1

Vocabulary Study

以下の①〜⑩の語（句）の意味をa.〜j.から選びましょう．そのうえで実際に発音を練習してみましょう．

① caution   a. 肥満
② hyperglycemia   b. 両側の
③ obesity   c. 糖尿病患者
④ bilateral   d. 疲れ果てた
⑤ exhausted   e. 分泌する
⑥ pancreas   f. 網膜症
⑦ secrete   g. 感覚，知覚
⑧ diabetic   h. 高血糖
⑨ sensation   i. 警告する
⑩ retinopathy   j. 膵臓

Mitsuo Mori is a 45-year-old system engineer. He has worked at a computer company for 17 years. His weight increased by 10 kilograms a year after he got the job, and his Body Mass Index surpassed 30 at the age of 30. At that time at a company periodical medical checkup, he was cautioned about hyperglycemia and obesity. However, he did not have any medical examination or treatment for 10 years after that.

He has suffered from dysesthesia on his bilateral fingertips for three years and felt exhausted. He has got tired very quickly even doing the clerical work. He has had difficulty in looking at documents on the computer, and finally he was admitted to the department of internal medicine at a hospital.

Mitsuo's pancreas did not secrete sufficient insulin, and the cells in his body did not take in enough glucose. He was diagnosed with type 2 diabetes mellitus, which more than 95 percent of Japanese diabetics suffer from. In his body, insulin did not function normally; therefore, the cells could not take in enough glucose, and he could not produce sufficient energy.

Kyoko Hibino, an occupational therapist with ten-year clinical experience, was put in charge of Mitsuo. After she listened to him about his work, she gave him a vision field test and a fingertip sensation test. He saw a small black spot moving and his vision was very blurred. He had developed myodesopsia and retinopathy, and he was in danger of losing his eyesight. He had lost almost all of the touch sensation of his fingers and the position sensation of his joints.

Kyoko instructed him to touch objects with the back of his hand in order to avoid getting injured. She told him to plug and unplug an electric appliance with the back of his hand facing the electric outlet. This is a strategy for quickly getting away from the outlet when his fingers are reactively flexed by an unexpected electric shock. Retinopathy, which he had developed, is the biggest cause of eyesight loss among adults. She told him that he should try not to hold his breath and strain himself to avoid an increase of the venous pressure in the retina.

He was instructed to undergo exercise therapy so that more insulin would be secreted, make the insulin function better, and help his muscular cells further take in glucose. He began to walk on the treadmill in the hospital for more than thirty minutes, one hour after he ate a meal prepared for diabetics.

Notes：**dysesthesia** 感覚異常.

Reading Comprehension

本文の内容に一致するものにはT（True），異なるものにはF（False）を記入しましょう．

① Mitsuo gained a lot of weight before he became a system engineer.　（　　）
② Mitsuo's Body Mass Index was just 30 at the age of 30.　（　　）
③ Mitsuo heard about hyperglycemia and obesity in a medical checkup.　（　　）
④ Mitsuo had some physical problems, and he was hospitalized.　（　　）
⑤ Kyoko worked for the clinic for ten years.　（　　）
⑥ Mitsuo's vision test and sensation test showed that he had serious problems.　（　　）
⑦ Kyoko told Mitsuo to touch his back with his fingers.　（　　）
⑧ Retinopathy can result in blindness.　（　　）
⑨ Mitsuo was advised to start medications to make his cells further take in glucose.　（　　）
⑩ Mitsuo walked for one hour after he ate a meal.　（　　）

パーツと語源で覚える医学用語

● **hyperglycemia** 高血糖（症）

　hyper-「過度の（over/excessive）」はギリシャ語由来の接頭辞．glycemia「血糖症」はギリシャ語由来の前部連結形 glyc(o)-「糖（sugar）」と後部連結形 -emia/-aemia「〜な血液を有する状態（blood condition）」からなる．

● **dysesthesia/dysaesthesia** 感覚異常

　dys- は「悪化（bad），困難な（difficult）」の意（Unit 3 を参照）．esthesia/aesthesia は「感覚能力，知覚力（sensitivity）」を表すギリシャ語由来の語彙．

● **diabetes mellitus** 真性糖尿病

　サイフォン（siphon）の意のギリシャ語 diabetes が語源．喉の渇きが激しくなり，いくら水を飲んでも尿が出てゆく病状に由来．さらに語義を遡るとギリシャ語 diabainein「通り過ぎる（go through）」に至る．dia-「〜を通って」+ bainein「行く」．後に，糖尿病患者の尿が蜂蜜のように甘いことが知られるようになりラテン語で「蜜のように甘い」を意味するラテン語 mellitus とあわせて diabetes mellitus が疾患名となった．

● **myodesopsia** 飛蚊症

　-opsia「〜視」はギリシャ語由来の後部連結形．ギリシャ語 muioeides「蚊のように（like a fly）」+ -opsia の構造．

● **retinopathy** 網膜症

　retin(o)- は「網膜（retina）」の意のラテン語由来の前部連結形．-pathy「病気（disease）」については Unit 3 を参照．

Reading 2

Vocabulary Study

以下の①~⑩の語（句）の意味を a.~j. から選びましょう．そのうえで実際に発音を練習してみましょう．

① density
② glucose
③ urine
④ metabolism
⑤ viscosity
⑥ arteriosclerosis
⑦ complication
⑧ dialysis
⑨ gangrene
⑩ hypoglycemic

a. ブドウ糖
b. 粘性
c. 血糖降下の，低血糖（症）の
d. 代謝
e. 壊疽
f. 合併症
g. 動脈硬化（症）
h. 濃度
i. 透析
j. 尿

    Diabetes Mellitus (DM) is characterized by continuous high density of glucose in the blood. Some people believe that DM is a disease in which sugar is found in the urine, but actually that is one of the symptoms of a high blood glucose level. Cells exposed to hyperglycemia have a poor function of glucose intake, and glucose which cannot be taken in by the cells adversely affects the kidneys that produce urine.

    Carbohydrates which we take in from meals are broken down into glucose in the small intestine and absorbed into the bloodstream. Protein and fat which are digested and broken down cause a rise in blood sugar. A hormone called insulin helps cells take in glucose from the blood to be used for energy in daily life. When insulin is not secreted by the pancreas or cannot act on cell membranes, cells have difficulty in taking in glucose and get little energy from the glucose metabolism. Therefore, the blood sugar level remains high.

    Hyperglycemia which engenders high viscosity in the blood may cause arteriosclerosis and bloodstream disorders. Retinopathy, nephropathy, and neuropathy are three major complications of diabetes. When these complications are aggravated, patients may suffer from loss of eyesight, renal failure that requires dialysis, and gangrene that can lead to amputation of lower limbs.

    The patients who do not show positive effects of diet therapy and exercise therapy for several months should start medications. Antidiabetic drugs include hypoglycemic drugs and insulin preparations. No matter what kind of medication the patients start, diet therapy and exercise therapy are required.

    In diet therapy, doctors decide the amount of meals relevant to the build and weight of the diabetics and their daily physical activity level. There are not any foods which the patients must not eat, but they have to be careful about what they eat. It is important to include a variety of foods and watch portion sizes.

They should have nutritionally well-balanced meals based on their weight and daily caloric requirements. They need to have healthy eating habits and manage their blood glucose.

In exercise therapy, exercise intensity and duration suitable for diabetic patients are considered, and appropriate exercises are prescribed. When they continue to do exercises and stimulate muscular cells, more glucose transporter type 4 (GLUT4) is expressed to the surface of muscle membranes to transport glucose, and muscles produce energy using glucose. Exercise is effective in lowering the blood glucose level, and exercise therapy enhances responsiveness of the muscles and the liver to insulin and promotes intake of glucose in the body.

> **Notes**: **carbohydrates** 炭水化物, **nephropathy** 腎臓病, **neuropathy** 神経障害, **renal failure** 腎不全, **insulin preparation** インスリン製剤.

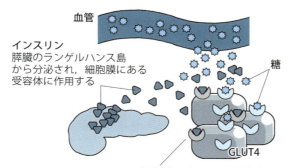

Comprehension Questions

以下の問いに英語で答えましょう．

① What is Diabetes Mellitus characterized by?
② What do cells exposed to hyperglycemia cause?
③ What happens to carbohydrates taken in our body?
④ Which organ produces insulin?
⑤ What happens when insulin is not secreted or cannot act on cell membranes?
⑥ Why can hyperglycemia cause arteriosclerosis?
⑦ In what cases is dialysis needed?
⑧ What kind of patients should begin to take medicines for diabetes?
⑨ What do doctors decide in diet therapy?
⑩ What is considered for diabetics in exercise therapy?

パーツと語源で覚える医学用語

● **arteriosclerosis** 動脈硬化（症）
　前部連結形 arteri(o)-「動脈（artery）」＋sclerosis「硬化症」．さらに sclerosis は scler(o)-「硬い（hard）」＋-osis「病的状態（abnormal condition）」の構造．いずれもギリシャ語由来の要素．

● **nephropathy** 腎臓病，**neuropathy** 神経障害
　nephr(o)- は「腎臓（kidney）」の意のギリシャ語由来の前部連結形．neur(o)-「神経（nerve），神経系（nervous system）」については Unit 9 の neurotransmitter を，-pathy「病気（disease）」については Unit 3 の arthropathy を参照．

● **dialysis** 透析
　ギリシャ語 *dialuein*「分ける（separate）」に由来．dia-「離れて，別個に（apart）」（Unit 3 を参照）＋-lysis「分解（disintegration）」＝dialysis「透析」．

● **hypoglycemic** 低血糖（症）の
　hypoglycemia「低血糖（症）」の形容詞形．接頭辞 hypo-「下の・不足の（below/deficient）」＋glycemia「血糖症」＝hypoglycemia「低血糖（症）」．glycemia については Reading 1 の hyperglycemia「高血糖（症）」の解説を参照．

Dictation

録音を聴いて空欄を埋め，各英文を完成させましょう．

① Some people believe that DM is (　　　　　　　　　　　　　　　　　　　),
but actually that is one of the symptoms of a high blood glucose level.

② (　　　　　　　　　　　　　　　　　　　) take in glucose from the blood
to be used for energy in daily life.

③ No (　　　　　　　　　　　　　　　　　　　), diet therapy and
exercise therapy are required.

Composition

日本語の意味に合うように〔　〕内の語（句）を並べ替えましょう．必要に応じて「,」を使用してください．

① その男性の体重は，年に5キロずつ増加して，昨年BMIは35を超えた．
The man's weight 〔 year, by, and, his, kilograms, a, five, surpassed, increased, BMI 〕 35 last year.

② 部長は，定期健康診断で肥満を警告された．
The department manager 〔 periodical, obesity, at, checkup, cautioned, a, about, was, medical 〕.

③ その患者は，小さな黒い点が動くのが見えたため，飛蚊症と診断された．
The patient 〔 with, a, he, was, because, saw, diagnosed, spot, myodesopsia, small black 〕 moving.

④ 私の叔父は，インスリンをさらに分泌させるために運動療法を指示された．
My uncle 〔 secreted, undergo, would be, instructed, to, was, so that, therapy, more insulin, exercise 〕.

⑤ 細胞に取り込まれることができないブドウ糖は，腎臓に悪影響を与える．
Glucose 〔 the kidneys, taken, cannot, which, in, cells, adversely affects, be, by 〕.

⑥ 私たちが食事で摂取する炭水化物は，ブドウ糖に分解されて，血液中に吸収される．
Carbohydrates 〔 meals, the bloodstream, in, broken, take, and, which, from, are, down, into, we, absorbed, glucose, into 〕.

⑦ インスリンという名のホルモンは，細胞が血液中のブドウ糖を取り込む手助けをする．
A hormone 〔 the blood, in, cells, insulin, take, from, called, glucose, helps 〕.

⑧ 糖尿病の患者は，透析が必要な腎不全をこうむるかもしれない．
Diabetic patients 〔 that, dialysis, failure, requires, from, suffer, renal, may 〕.

⑨ 食事療法の効果を示さなかった人たちは，薬物療法を開始した．
Those 〔 therapy, not, positive, show, medications, diet, did, of, started, who, effects 〕.

⑩ どのような薬物療法を彼らが開始しても，食事療法と運動療法は不可欠である．
〔 they, of, no, start, kind, matter, what, medication 〕, it is vital to have diet therapy and exercise therapy.

Medical Terms

第Ⅱ部のリスト（表1～3）を参考にA群の語彙の意味を調べたうえで，それらを用いてB群の空欄〔1〕～〔15〕を埋めましょう．

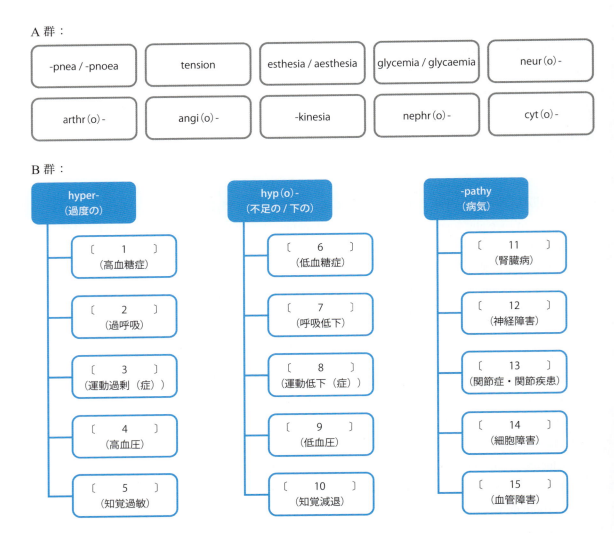

Let's try!

　In Reading 1, the diabetic patient began to walk on the treadmill in the hospital. What other exercises are recommended for diabetics by doctors and therapists?　Discuss the question in groups.

Unit 13
COPD（慢性閉塞性肺疾患）

　COPD（慢性閉塞性肺疾患）は chronic obstructive pulmonary disease の略で，煙草の煙に代表される有毒物質を長時間吸入することで生じる肺の炎症が原因の慢性呼吸器疾患の1つです．主な症状は咳，痰，息切れなどですが，重症化すると呼吸不全に陥ることもあり，2020年までに全世界の死亡原因の第3位になるとも推測されています．予防には禁煙と同時に肺機能検査などによる早期発見が欠かせません．

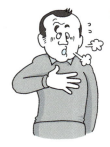

動くと息切れがする．

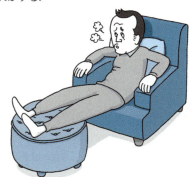

息切れを避けるために動かなくなる（身体活動量の低下）．

体力，筋力の低下．さらに動かなくなる．息切れも強くなる．

症状悪化

Reading 1

Vocabulary Study

以下の①〜⑩の語（句）の意味を a.〜j. から選びましょう．そのうえで実際に発音を練習してみましょう．

① obstructive　　　　　　　a. 咳
② shortness of breath　　　　b. 内科医
③ cough　　　　　　　　　　c. 吸い込む
④ disturb　　　　　　　　　d. 妨害する
⑤ sputum　　　　　　　　　e. 閉塞性の
⑥ internist　　　　　　　　　f. 息切れ
⑦ inhale　　　　　　　　　　g.（息を）吐き出す
⑧ exhale　　　　　　　　　　h. 痰
⑨ abdominal breathing　　　 i. 禁煙外来
⑩ smoking cessation clinic　　j. 腹式呼吸

Hiroshi Kimura is a high-school mathematics teacher. He is 55 years old and has been working for more than 30 years in Kagoshima. Teaching young students has been giving him valuable experiences, and he loves his job; however, his job is also a source of stress and pressure. He is a typical heavy smoker and has been smoking 30 cigarettes a day for more than 20 years. Although he understands that quitting smoking would be better for his health, he has failed whenever he has tried to quit.

When he was young, he often enjoyed hiking and skiing. However, for the last several years, he has not exercised and has started experiencing shortness of breath while walking up and down stairs. In addition, he began coughing at night, which disturbed his sleep. Furthermore, after smoking, he started producing sputum, which became cream in color. Therefore, Hiroshi finally went to see an internist and was diagnosed with chronic obstructive pulmonary disease (COPD). The doctor instructed him to stop smoking as soon as possible, to undergo lung function testing and to attend rehabilitation under the instruction of a physical therapist.

Takayuki Nagai, one of the physical therapists at the hospital where Hiroshi visited, evaluated Hiroshi's physical function by conducting several tests including spirometry. Spirometry measures how much air can be inhaled and exhaled and how fast air can move into and out of the lungs. The test results confirmed several factors contributing to COPD. The flexibility of the rib (thoracic) cage was decreased. The percentage of the forced expiratory volume in one second (FEV1), which is a measure of the greatest volume of air that can be exhaled in the first second of a breath, was low. The 6-minute walking test result was only 300 m (the average for an elderly individual is approximately 500 to 550 m) and the SpO_2 of 90% was lower than the standard volume. These results showed a decrease in his exercise tolerance.

Takayuki instructed Hiroshi how to breathe more easily when he had difficulty in breathing, i.e., breathing out twice as long as breathing in and trying abdominal breathing. He also instructed him on stretching exercises of the rib cage, training of the muscles involved in breathing and the lower limbs, and ways to walk in order to train his whole body. Lastly, he introduced the concept of pursed-lip breathing, which means breathing out with pursed lips.

Hiroshi tried these recommended ways of breathing every time he walked up and down stairs. He also took time to attend rehabilitation. Surprisingly, he felt that his breathing was easier. He recognized how breathing affected his daily life and finally decided to quit smoking completely. Therefore, he is now visiting a smoking cessation clinic.

Notes: **spirometry** 肺活量測定, **rib (thoracic) cage** 胸郭, **FEV1** 1秒量, **SpO_2** 動脈血酸素飽和度, **exercise tolerance** 運動耐容能, **pursed-lip breathing** 口すぼめ呼吸.

Reading Comprehension

本文の内容に一致するものにはT（True），異なるものにはF（False）を記入しましょう．

① Hiroshi does not like teaching. （　　）

② Hiroshi has been smoking for more than 20 years. （　　）

③ Because Hiroshi knew that smoking was bad for his health, he succeeded in quitting. （　　）

④ Hiroshi experienced shortness of breath while hiking and skiing. （　　）

⑤ In addition to being short of breath, Hiroshi coughed at night. （　　）

⑥ From the result of the spirometry test, Takayuki noticed Hiroshi's lung function had been declining. （　　）

⑦ The result of Hiroshi's 6-minute walking test was better than average. （　　）

⑧ Abdominal breathing, breathing out twice as long as breathing in, and pursed-lip breathing are helpful for COPD patients. （　　）

⑨ Stretching exercises and muscle training are not required as forms of rehabilitation for COPD patients. （　　）

⑩ Hiroshi decided to stop smoking after he tried what the physical therapist recommended. （　　）

パーツと語源で覚える医学用語

● **pulmonary** 肺の

　Unit 10 を参照．

● **disease** 病気

　Unit 9 を参照．

● **spirometry** 肺活量測定

　spir(o)-「呼吸（respiration）」はラテン語 *spirare*「呼吸する（breathe）」に由来する前部連結形．-metry「測定法（術）（学）（measurement）」はギリシャ語由来の後部連結形．-meter で終わる器具名に対応する（例：spirometer「肺活量計」）．

● **abdominal** 腹部の

　abdomen(o)-「腹部（abdomen）」の意のラテン語由来の前部連結形．-al「〜の」は形容詞をつくる接尾辞．

● **inhale** 吸い込む

　接頭辞 in- は「中へ（into）」の意．ラテン語 *inhalare*「吸い込む」に由来．in-「中へ」+ *halare*「呼吸する（breathe）」．

● **exhale** （息を）吐き出す

　接頭辞 ex- は「外に（out）」の意．ラテン語 *exhalare*「息を吐き出す」に由来．ex-「外に」+ *halare*「呼吸する（breathe）」．

Reading 2

Vocabulary Study

以下の①～⑩の語（句）の意味をa.～j.から選びましょう．そのうえで実際に発音を練習してみましょう．

① interfere　　　　　a. さらすこと
② vital capacity　　　b. 気道
③ exposure　　　　　c. 炎症
④ toxic　　　　　　　d. 早期発見
⑤ pollution　　　　　e. 栄養に関する
⑥ inflammation　　　f. 汚染
⑦ airway　　　　　　g. 摂取
⑧ nutritional　　　　h. 肺活量
⑨ intake　　　　　　i. 妨害する
⑩ early detection　　j. 有毒な

　COPD is a common chronic lung disease that interferes with normal breathing. When the forced vital capacity (FVC) declines, it is known as chronic restrictive pulmonary disease (CRPD). When the percentage of the FEV1 declines, it is known as chronic obstructive pulmonary disease. The most common symptoms of COPD are shortness of breath, abnormal sputum, and chronic cough. Daily activities, such as walking up and down stairs, may become very difficult as the condition gradually worsens.

　The primary cause of COPD is tobacco smoking either through direct tobacco use or second-hand smoke. Indoor and outdoor air pollution and dust and chemicals at work are also major risk factors of COPD. Heavy exposure to these toxic substances damages alveoli, causes inflammation of the airways, and contributes to COPD.

　COPD is confirmed by a test known as spirometry. Spirometry measures the amount of air a person can breathe out and the amount of time it takes to do so. Because 75-80% of FVC normally comes out in the first second, an FEV1/FVC ratio of less than 70%, along with symptoms of COPD, can confirm the diagnosis. COPD is not curable; however, it is treatable, and its progression can be delayed. It is essential to stop smoking in order to reduce the risk factors. Various forms of treatment can help decrease the symptoms and improve quality of life (QOL), including medication, breathing exercises, therapeutic exercises, and nutritional instruction.

　Regarding breathing exercises, abdominal breathing and breathing out longer than breathing in are the basic recommendations. Stretching up both arms when breathing in and dropping them down when breathing out also help to broaden the rib cage. Regarding therapeutic exercises, walking and regular training of the muscles involved in breathing and the lower limbs improve the tolerance of the whole body.

In underweight COPD patients, increasing caloric intake can lead to improvements in COPD symptoms. Currently, pulmonary rehabilitation (PR) covers almost all of the above therapeutic methods that are used in the treatment of COPD. PR involves a long-term commitment from the patient and a team of health care providers including doctors, nurses, physical therapists, occupational therapists, dietitians, social workers, and so on.

   A survey conducted by the Ministry of Health, Labour and Welfare showed that in Japan, more than 16,000 people died of COPD in 2014, and that the number of deaths has been increasing and will continue to increase. Globally, more than 3 million people died of COPD in 2012. COPD is not curable but is preventable. Therefore prevention by decreasing tobacco use and air pollution as well as early detection of the disease is the best approach.

> **Notes**：FVC 努力肺活量，chronic restrictive pulmonary disease (CRPD) 慢性拘束性肺疾患，alveoli 肺胞 (alveolus の複数形), pulmonary rehabilitation 呼吸リハビリテーション．

Comprehension Questions
以下の問いに英語で答えましょう．
① What are the common symptoms of COPD?
② What is the primary cause of COPD?
③ How do smoking and air pollution cause COPD?
④ What kind of test is conducted to diagnose COPD?
⑤ What is the most important approach to reduce the risk factors of COPD?
⑥ How should COPD patients breathe?
⑦ Why are walking and regular muscle training recommended for COPD patients?
⑧ If a COPD patient is underweight, what is necessary as treatment?
⑨ What do you call the rehabilitation including various forms of teatment for COPD patients?
⑩ According to the survey by the Ministry of Health, Labour and Welfare, how many people died of COPD globally in 2012?

パーツと語源で覚える医学用語

- **abnormal** 異常な
  接頭辞 ab-「〜から離れている（away from）」+ normal「正常な」.

- **alveoli**「肺胞」の複数形
  単数形は alveolus．前部連結形 alveol(o)-「肺胞/歯槽（alveolus）」はラテン語 *alveus*「小さな空洞」に由来．

- **diagnosis** 診断
  Unit 3 を参照．

- **dietitian/dietician** 栄養士
  -ician は「専門家（specialist）」の意のフランス語由来の接尾辞．-itian も同じ意味の異形．diet「食物（food）」+ -itian/-ician「専門家（specialist）」．

Dictation

録音を聴いて空欄を埋め，各英文を完成させましょう．

① The therapist （　　　　　　　　　　　　　　　　　　　　　　　　　　）．
② The average of （　　　　　　　　　　　　　　　　　　　　　　　　） is approximately 500 to 550 m.
③ The common symptoms of COPD are （　　　　　　　　　　　　　　　　　）．

Composition

日本語の意味に合うように〔　〕内の語（句）を並べ替えましょう．必要に応じて「,」を使用してください．

① 彼は禁煙を試みるたびいつも失敗してきた．

He has failed 〔 he, tried, smoking, whenever, has, to quit 〕．

② 私の母は医師と理学療法士の指示のもとリハビリテーションに励んでいる．

My mother 〔 of a doctor, rehabilitation programs, attends, the instruction, under 〕 and a physical therapist.

③ 療法士は祖母にもっと楽に階段の昇り降りをする方法を教えてくれた．

The therapist instructed 〔 how, walk up and down, my grandmother, to, stairs, more easily 〕．

④ 痛みのために，駅まで歩くのに予想の3倍の時間がかかった．

Because of pain,〔 as long as, took, three times, I had expected, to the station, walking 〕．

⑤ 手首をきつく締めると血液の循環が妨げられる．

A tight belt for 〔 will interfere, the wrist, with, circulation, of the blood 〕．

⑥ 右手でも左手でもどちらでもよいので棒をつかんでください．

Please 〔 your right, grab, with, either, or left hand, the bar 〕．

⑦ 長時間汚染された大気に触れると，気道に炎症を起こすかもしれない．

Heavy 〔 to, may cause, polluted air, inflammation, exposure 〕 of the airways.

⑧ 定期的にリハビリテーションをすることで体全体の耐久性がよくなり，COPDの治療につながる．

Regular rehabilitation can〔 improvements, and cure, of the whole body, lead to, of the tolerance 〕 for COPD.

⑨ 呼吸リハビリテーションは，COPD治療に必要なほとんどすべての療法を含んでいる．

Pulmonary rehabilitation 〔 all of, covers, almost, in, the therapeutic methods, required 〕 the treatment of COPD.

⑩ 厚生労働省の調査によると，COPDによる死亡者数は年々増加している．

A survey conducted by the Ministry of Health, Labour and Welfare 〔 the number of deaths, has, shows, been increasing, that, by COPD 〕 year by year.

Medical Terms

第Ⅱ部のリスト（表1〜3）を参考に，下記の前部連結形を用いて医学用語をつくり，空欄〔1〕〜〔8〕を埋めましょう．

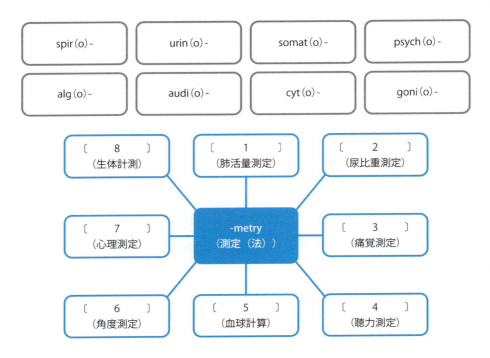

Let's try!

If some of your friends are smokers, how would you persuade them to quit?

Make a dialog between a smoker and a friend who wants to persuade him or her to quit smoking with your partner.

Unit 14
Cerebral Palsy（脳性麻痺）

　脳性麻痺とは，胎児が体内にいるときから生後4週までの間に起きた，脳の何らかの障害による運動の異常を意味します．年齢とともに進行する麻痺や，単に発達が遅れている状態は脳性麻痺とは呼びません．現代の医学では完治することができないため，障がいがあっても姿勢，運動，摂食，発語などをうまくコントロールしていけるよう，治療やトレーニングを行います．理学療法，作業療法，言語聴覚療法を有効に利用し患者の生活の質を少しでも高めることが肝要です．

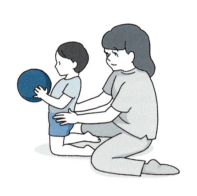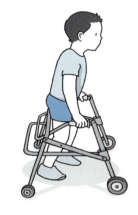

脳性麻痺児のトレーニングの様子

Reading 1

Vocabulary Study

以下の①〜⑩の語（句）の意味を a.〜j. から選びましょう．そのうえで実際に発音を練習してみましょう．

① wheelchair　　　　　　　　a. 算数
② arithmetic　　　　　　　　 b. カルテ
③ junior　　　　　　　　　　 c. 大学3年生
④ clinical practice　　　　　　d. 主訴
⑤ medical records（chart）　　e. 〜を感動させる
⑥ supervisor　　　　　　　　 f. 車椅子
⑦ gymnasium　　　　　　　　g. 指導教官
⑧ disability　　　　　　　　　h. 臨床実習
⑨ impress　　　　　　　　　 i. 体育館
⑩ chief complaint　　　　　　j. 障がい

Takashi Ito is an 11-year-old boy with cerebral palsy. Because he has paralysis in both lower limbs, he was diagnosed as having diplegia and uses a wheelchair. For five years, he has been studying at a special support school with other students with cerebral palsy. He is good at arithmetic but his favorite activity is playing baseball after school.

Haruto Tajima is a junior, majoring in physical therapy. He began four weeks of clinical practice at the special support school this week. Before beginning, he attempted to obtain information regarding Takashi, whom he was in charge of. Takashi's medical records showed that he could not stand by himself and used a wheelchair, and that he loved playing baseball. Haruto got interested in how children with cerebral palsy play baseball.

On the first day of clinical practice, although Haruto met Takashi, Takashi did not provide any detailed information regarding his health. On the advice of his practice supervisor, Haruto had a good opportunity to observe the after-school activities in the school gymnasium. It was the first time he had observed people with disabilities playing baseball. Surprisingly, several students with physical impairment were cheerfully playing baseball, and appearing to enjoy moving. He carefully observed how they were playing. Some fielders were sitting with two legs bent on each side. Others were defending in their wheelchairs. A pitcher in a wheelchair rolled the ball to the batter. The batter, sitting with two legs bent on each side, swung the bat, hit the ball, and began crawling on his hands and knees toward the first base ; that was Takashi. His enthusiastic appearance truly impressed Haruto.

According to the supervisor, the school has used this method of playing baseball for more than 10 years. A sitting position with two legs bent on each side is not recommended, because it may cause dislocation of the hip joint and incorrect posture, contribute to scoliosis and result in restrictive ventilator impairment. However, the supervisor said that they allowed the students to adopt this posture only when playing baseball to enjoy it more.

The following day, Haruto and Takashi enjoyed talking about baseball a lot, and through their conversation, Haruto learned what Takashi's chief complaint was. Although it is basically quite difficult to understand a child's chief complaint in detail from an interview, talking about baseball helped him very much. Takashi's complaint was that he was getting bigger physically and his muscles were stronger ; however, as his bones were growing faster than his muscles, the muscle tone of his legs was being strained ; therefore, his body was stiff, making it difficult to smoothly play baseball.

Haruto is wondering how he can assist Takashi to enjoy baseball. Enjoying something increases a patient's quality of life. Being confident that good rehabilitation can help to achieve this, Haruto will learn a lot through clinical practice.

Notes : diplegia 両麻痺, special support school 特別支援学校, sitting with two legs bent on each side 割り座, scoliosis 脊柱側弯（症）, restrictive ventilator impairment 拘束性換気障害, muscle tone（tonus）筋緊張.

Reading Comprehension

本文の内容に一致するものには T（True），異なるものには F（False）を記入しましょう．

① Takashi was paralyzed because of an accident at school. （　　）

② Because he can walk by himself, Takashi does not require a wheelchair. （　　）

③ Takashi likes to play baseball after school. （　　）

④ Before he began clinical practice, Haruto was so busy that he did not prepare for it at all. （　　）

⑤ On the first day of clinical practice, Haruto could talk a lot with Takashi regarding his health. （　　）

⑥ Watching people with disabilities playing baseball was impressive for Haruto. （　　）

⑦ Sitting with two legs bent on each side is a recommended posture for students with physical impairments. （　　）

⑧ Thanks to talking about baseball, Haruto was able to understand Takashi's concern. （　　）

⑨ As Takashi is growing, his body is becoming flexible. （　　）

⑩ One of the most important targets of rehabilitation is to increase the quality of life of the patients. （　　）

パーツと語源で覚える医学用語

● **cerebral** 脳の
Unit 5 の cerebrovascular を参照．

● **paralysis** 麻痺
Unit 7 を参照．

● **diplegia** 両麻痺
di- は「2（two/double）」の意のギリシャ語由来の接頭辞．-plegia「麻痺（paralysis）」については Unit 7 の quadriplegia/tetraplegia を参照．

● **scoliosis** 脊柱側弯（症）
ギリシャ語 *skolios*「屈曲（bent）」に由来．-osis「病的状態」については Unit 4 の osteoporosis を参照．

Reading 2

Vocabulary Study

以下の①～⑩の語（句）の意味を a.～j. から選びましょう．そのうえで実際に発音を練習してみましょう．

① pregnancy　　　　　　a. 運動麻痺
② labor　　　　　　　　b. 変形
③ delivery　　　　　　　c. 出産
④ motor paralysis　　　　d. 分娩の過程
⑤ crutch　　　　　　　　e. 進行性の
⑥ progressive　　　　　　f. 知力（知能）の
⑦ fatal　　　　　　　　　g. 専門職間の
⑧ deformation　　　　　　h. 致命的な
⑨ intellectual　　　　　　i. 妊娠
⑩ interprofessional　　　　j. 松葉づえ

　Cerebral palsy (CP) refers to a group of disorders that affect muscle movement and the ability to move which is caused by brain damage, which occurs before four weeks of age. Some of the main causes of CP are complications during pregnancy, labor, or delivery. Paralysis that develops because of brain damage after four weeks of age is not considered to be CP.

　Although CP refers to motor paralysis, the symptoms of physical impairment vary among individuals. It can affect the arms, legs, face, several limbs, or all of these. Therefore, some patients only have limited impairments, whereas others are unable to walk, stand still, or even crawl or roll over, and they require various assisting tools, such as crutches and wheelchairs, and total nursing care. Based on the condition, CP is divided into 3 types: spastic, ataxic, and athetoid. Furthermore, CP can result in additional medical disorders such as respiratory problems (e.g., restrictive ventilator impairment), dysphagia, and speech or communication problems.

　CP permanently affects body movement and muscle conditions, but it is not progressive or fatal. Most children with CP grow up to be adults. Various forms of treatment and therapy are available to improve the patients' capabilities and help increase their independence. Although the therapeutic measures applied to the patients depend on how serious their disorder is, there are some common and important matters to remember as follows:

1. You need to prevent deformation of the joints particularly during the growing years because bones grow faster than muscles, and this can greatly affect the movement of the joints.
2. You need to check the posture of the patients particularly during the elementary and junior high school years and use assisting tools such as wheelchairs, if necessary.

3. You need to carefully observe the development of restrictive ventilator impairment because of scoliosis, which often occurs because of being in an unnatural posture for a long time.
4. You need to prevent patients from lying in bed in the same posture or sitting with two legs bent on each side for a long time because these may cause dislocation of the hip joint.
5. You need to provide treatments and therapies for the whole body to prevent decline in total physical strength because of inflexible joints, limited physical activity, and weakened muscle strength.

In the absence of severe intellectual or physical disorders, children with CP may attend schools for regular education. However, most of them have to undergo extensive rehabilitation and receive special support education. Because their ability to move is severely restricted, they require some type of nursing care throughout their lives. That is why interprofessional cooperation is necessary to find and apply good and effective educational and therapeutic measures to increase their independence and quality of life.

Notes：spastic 痙直型の，ataxic 運動失調型の，athetoid アテトーゼ型の（不随意運動型の）

Comprehension Questions
以下の問いに英語で答えましょう．
① What does cerebral palsy (CP) refer to?
② What are some of the main causes of CP?
③ Do all the patients with CP have similar disorders?
④ What are the typical assisting tools for CP patients?
⑤ What are the three types of CP?
⑥ Besides motor paralysis, what types of disorders do patients with CP tend to have?
⑦ How does deformation of the joints occur in patients with CP?
⑧ Why should CP patients avoid lying in bed in the same posture for a long time?
⑨ Why are treatments and therapies for the whole body required?
⑩ Why should we have interprofessional cooperation for children with CP?

パーツと語源で覚える医学用語

- **ataxic** 運動失調の（を伴う）

  ataxia「運動失調（症）」の形容詞形．ギリシャ語由来．*a-*「無（without）」+ *taxis*「秩序（order）」の構造で，元来は不規則性，無秩序の意．

- **athetoid** アテトーゼ型の（不随意運動型の）・アテトーシス（**athetosis**）様の

  ギリシャ語 *athetos*（without position）+ -osis「病的状態」．

- **dysphagia** 嚥下障害

  Unit 9 を参照．

- **deformation** 変形

  ラテン語 *deformare* に由来．*de-*「下降，分離，悪化」+ *forma*「形」= deform「〜の形を損なう」．

- **interprofessional** 専門職間の

  inter-「間・相互の」と professional「専門職の」の合成語．

Dictation

録音を聴いて空欄を埋め，各英文を完成させましょう．

① Cerebral palsy（CP）refers to a（　　　　　　　　　　　　　　　　　　　　　）

　　that occurs before, during, or immediately after birth.

② The therapeutic measures（　　　　　　　　　　　　　　　　　　　　　　　　）．

③ Most children（　　　　　　　　　　　　　　　　　　　）and receive special

　　support education.

Composition

日本語の意味に合うように〔 〕内の語（句）を並べ替えましょう．必要に応じて「，」を使用してください．

① 私は脳性麻痺の患者を担当している．

　　I〔 am, cerebral palsy, of, charge, a patient, in, with 〕．

② 先生のアドバイスのおかげで，オーストラリアに留学する好機を得た．

　　I had〔 the teacher's advice, to study, a good opportunity, in Australia, on 〕．

③ 療法士の笑顔は患者の緊張をほぐしてくれる．

　　A〔 the therapist's face, smile, on, can, patients, relax 〕．

④ 実習指導者は，学生がその患者に面談することを認めてくれた．

　　The clinical supervisor〔 the student, to have, allowed, with the patient, an interview 〕．

⑤ 結果として，彼女の筋の動きは向上した．

　　Her〔 improved, a result, muscle movement, was, as 〕．

⑥ 1人で歩ける患者もいれば，寝返りが困難な患者もいる．

　　Some patients can walk by themselves,〔 have, whereas, rolling over, difficulty, in, others 〕．

⑦ 脳性麻痺とは，生後4週間以内に起きた脳の障害が原因の運動機能障害のことである．

　　Cerebral palsy〔 caused, refers to, disorders, of motor function, by brain damage 〕before four weeks of age.

⑧ 嚥下障害やことばの障害といった機能障害は患者それぞれで現れ方が異なる．

　　Disorders〔 one patient, dysphagia and speech problems, such as, to another, vary, from 〕．

⑨ その疾患の原因は3つの要因に分けられる．

　　The causes〔 divided, of, the disease, are, three factors, into 〕．

⑩ 不自然な姿勢を長く続けると関節の変形が起きやすい．

　　Keeping〔 may cause, of the joints, an unnatural posture, for a long time, deformation 〕．

Unit 14　Cerebral Palsy（脳性麻痺）

Medical Terms

第Ⅱ部のリスト（表1～3）を参考に，次の連結形を組み合わせて①～⑩の病名をつくりましょう．必要があれば同じ連結形を何度使っても構いません．

angi(o)-	ureter(o)-	por(o)-	arteri(o)-
py(o)-	oste(o)-	neur(o)-	nephr(o)-
sten(o)-	scler(o)-	bronch(o)-	necr(o)-
-osis			

① 壊死　　　　　（　　　　　　　　）
② 骨粗鬆症　　　（　　　　　　　　）
③ 腎臓症　　　　（　　　　　　　　）
④ 動脈硬化症　　（　　　　　　　　）
⑤ 神経症　　　　（　　　　　　　　）
⑥ 化膿（症）　　（　　　　　　　　）
⑦ 血管狭窄（症）（　　　　　　　　）
⑧ 気管支狭窄　　（　　　　　　　　）
⑨ 尿管狭窄症　　（　　　　　　　　）
⑩ 尿管化膿症　　（　　　　　　　　）

Let's try!

　If you were Haruto, what could you do to help resolve Takashi's complaints? Talk with your partner in English.

第Ⅱ部　医学用語の学習

語源とパーツによる学習方法

　ここではリハビリテーションを志す学生に限らず，看護学をはじめとするほかの医療分野の皆様にもご活用いただけるように，医療全般にわたり専門用語を提示しています．解説や練習問題の構成にあたっては皆さんが医学英語の独学をしている状況を想定し，学習者にとって極力わかりやすい説明を心がけました．第Ⅱ部を医学用語学習の参考書としてご活用ください．

　また，学習の便宜をはかるため，巻末に接辞と連結形のリスト（**表1**：全要素のアルファベット順，**表2**：接頭辞と前部連結形の分野別，**表3**：接尾辞と後部連結形の分野別）を用意し，本書全体の医学用語に関する練習問題の学習に活用できるように構成されています．とくに，**表1**は医学用語のパーツとなる語頭と語末の接辞と連結形を一括し，アルファベット順に配列しています．医学用語学習の際の辞書代わりとしてご活用いただけます．

1. はじめに：英語における学術用語の由来

　医学用語の多くは古典ギリシャ語に由来します．地中海一帯を支配し，ローマ帝国を築いたローマ人は古代ギリシャ文明を受け継ぎ，多くのギリシャ語の学術用語がローマ字化されてラテン語に取り入れられました．ギリシャ語起源の学術用語・医学用語を抱えたラテン語はローマ帝国の繁栄とともにヨーロッパの共通言語となりますが，このラテン語から多くの語彙が英語へと借入されます．とくに，初期近代英語期（1450〜1650 年頃）は芸術・学問が隆盛を極めたルネサンス期に重なり，大量の語彙が古典ギリシャ語・ラテン語から英語に流入しました．この時期の借入語は古典ラテン語から直接借入されたため，硬い語感を持つものが多いのが特徴です．この時期，学者たちによってあまりに大量の借入語が用いられたため，これらの難解な語は inkhorn term（インク壺語：inkhorn は「角製のインク入れ」のこと．ラテン語やギリシャ語から取り入れた博学を気取った難解な言葉を指す）と呼ばれ揶揄されたほどです．現在，ラテン語は母（国）語としては話されていませんが，その語彙は英単語の中に取り込まれ，生き続けているのです．

　医学用語をはじめとして，科学専門用語の多くはギリシャ語やラテン語の単語に由来する語根（root：単語の意味の基本となる部分で，それ以上分解不可能な単位）と呼ばれる要素を含む連結形（combining form）が，ほかの語，連結形・接辞と結合することで構成されています．そして，これらの科学用語の多くはギリシャ語・ラテン語由来の要素を含んではいますが，現代になってからの造語であるため，新古典複合語（neo-classical compound）と呼ばれます．たとえば，quadriplegia（四肢麻痺）という語はラテン語由来の quadri- とギリシャ語由来の -plegia という 2 つの古典的連結形から成り立っていますが，quadriplegia という語自体は 1920 年代の造語です．このようにギリシャ語やラテン語に由来する連結形を用いて，次々と新しい学問用語がつくられているのです．医学用語を効率よく学習するためには，(a) 語の構造を理解すること，(b) 連結形や接辞（affix）と呼ばれる構成要素の語源的意味を理解することが重要です．じつは，医学用語は大変シンプルな構造であり，簡単なルールに従って組み立てられています．では，順を追って医学用語を学習していきましょう．

2. 医学用語の基礎知識

2.1　医学用語の構造と意味

　個々の語（word）はさらに小さな意味を持つパーツに分解することができます．gastrotomy（胃切開）という用語を例に，その内部構造をみてみましょう．語頭の gastr- の部分はギリシャ語に由来し，「胃」を意味します．語末の -tomy の部分もギリシャ語由来で「切開」を意味します．gastr- と -tomy 間にある -o- は連結母音（combining vowel）と呼ばれ，2 つの要素をつなげて発音しやすくするものです．「胃」+「切開」=「胃切開」という極めて理解しやすい構造になっています．

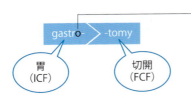

図1　gastrotomy（胃切開）の構造
ICF：initial combining form, FCF：final combining form.

同様にgastroscope「胃鏡・胃カメラ」はgastr(o)-と-scope（〜を見る器械・〜鏡）に分解できます．gastrotomyと似た単語でgastrectomyがありますが，-ectomyもギリシャ語由来で「切除」を意味し，gastrectomyは「胃切除」を意味します．

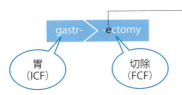

図2　gastrectomy（胃切除）の構造

gastrotomyやgastrectomyは2つの要素から成る用語ですが，もっと複雑な例をみてみましょう．
　otorhinolaryngologyという語をはじめて目にした人は，綴りも複雑で長く，どう発音してよいか戸惑うのではないでしょうか．発音はともかく，意味は何でしょう．語末が-logyで終わっているから何かの学問分野であると推測された方は，医学用語学習に必要な基礎力が充分あります．この語はot(o)-「耳」，rhin(o)-「鼻」，laryng(o)-「喉頭」，-logy「学問」という4つのパーツからなり，「耳鼻咽喉科（学）」を意味します．なお，図1〜3で示された各用語を構成する個々の要素は連結形（CF：combining form）と呼ばれますが，辞書によっては接辞（affix）として分類している場合もあります．

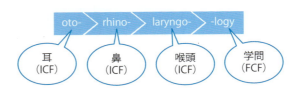

図3　otorhinolaryngology（耳鼻咽喉科学）の構造

　一見難しそうに見える医学用語ですが，語よりも小さな意味を持つ要素に注目し，各構成単位の意味に基づいて語全体の意味を理解することにより，語彙学習が効率化されるとともに，より深いレベルで処理されるため記憶保持が促進されることは間違いありません．医学用語の学習においては，丸暗記ではなく，理解して覚える楽しさを感じてください．では，語よりも小さな単位に分解し，構造を理解するために必要な基礎知識を以下で学習しましょう．

2.2 接辞（affix）と連結形（combining form）

図1のgastrotomyや図2のgastrectomyを構成するgastr(o)-，-tomy，-ectomyは連結形（combining form）と呼ばれることはすでに述べましたが，これらは接辞（affix）とはどう違うのでしょうか．接辞とは語（word）や語根（root：語の中核的意味を表し，それ以上分析できない要素）の前後に添加して，語の意味を変更・修正したり，語の文法的特性を表す要素です．図4のepigastric（上腹部の）という形容詞を例に接辞の特性を考えてみましょう．

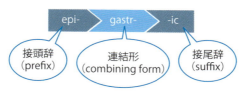

図4　epigastric（上腹部の）の構造

> **接辞（affix）：**
> 語頭要素である接頭辞（prefix）と語末要素の接尾辞（suffix）をあわせて接辞（affix）と呼ぶ．接辞は独立語としては存在しない形式（拘束形式：bound form）であり，語根（root）となる連結形（combining form）や語（word）の前後に添加して語義の変更，修正，意味の追加，文法的特性等の表示を行う．通常，接頭辞と接尾辞の連結はできない．また，接頭辞と語根との連結に際して連結母音は用いない．

epigastricという語の中核はgastr-（胃）という連結形で，語根（root）になっています．この語根の前後に「～の上，外側」の意の接頭辞epi-と「～の」の意味を示す形容詞をつくる接尾辞-icが添加しています．接辞と呼ばれるepi-や-icのような要素は，語の中核をなす語根やほかの語に添加して存在できる言語形式ですが，それら単独では存在できません．このように単独で用いられることのない言語形式は拘束形式（bound form）と呼ばれます．また接辞の特徴として，接辞どうしの結合，つまり，接頭辞と接尾辞の結合は通常できないという点があげられます．一般的な単語を例にあげると，international（国際的な）のinter-（～の間の，相互に）や-al（～の）などがすぐに思い浮かぶ接頭辞，接尾辞の例です．

では，連結形と接辞とはどのような違いがあるのでしょうか．すでに図1～3において，連結形の具体例をみてきました．連結形と接辞には共通点があります．なぜなら，連結形も独立して存在することができない拘束形式だからです．また，語頭に位置するgastr-のような要素は前部連結形（ICF：initial combining form），語末に位置する-tomyのような要素は後部連結形（FCF：final combining form）と呼ばれますので，この点も接頭辞，接尾辞に似ています．じつは，辞書によっては連結形と接辞の区別をせず，両者をまとめて接辞として表示しているものもあります．しかし，詳しい辞書になると接辞と連結形を区別する場合が多いようです．両者の違いに着目しつつ，連結形の特徴を箇条書きにしてみます．

連結形（combining form）の特徴：

(1) 連結形はギリシャ語，ラテン語に由来し，接辞と同様に独立語としては存在しない形式（拘束形式：bound form）である．
(2) 接頭辞と接尾辞は通常，互いに連結することができないが，前部連結形と後部連結形の連結は可能である（例，gastrotomy：gastro- + -tomy）．
(3) 連結形は語や連結形だけでなく，接辞と結びつくことが可能である（例，gastric：gastr- + -ic）．
(4) 一般的傾向として連結形は接辞よりも意味がより具体的である（語彙情報の密度が高い）．
(5) 一般的傾向として連結形どうしの連結の関係は等位的であり，どれが語の中心的意味を成しているとは決めがたい場合が多い（例，gastrotomy「胃切開」：gastro-「胃」+ -tomy「切開」）．
(6) 前部連結形が語末要素（後部連結形や接尾辞）と結びつく場合，語末要素の先頭が子音の場合は通常，連結母音 -o- が使われる．一方，接辞と語根との連結には連結母音は現れない．
(7) 連結形は語形成上の生産性が比較的に低いが（結びつく要素が限られてくる），典型的な接辞は生産性が比較的に高く，多くの要素と結びついて新語を生み出せる（生産性が高い接辞の例：inter-「相互の」, intra-「内の」, hypo-「下の・不足の」, hyper-「過度の」）．

しかしながら，これらの特徴はあくまでも一般的傾向であり，両者の区分に絶対的な基準はなく，上記で述べた特徴の例外が存在します．連結形を接辞の一部として扱う辞書が多いのも，それに起因するのでしょう．また，連結形と接辞を区別している辞書の間でも同一の形式の分類に違いがみられる場合があることは，両者の違いが相対的なものであり，絶対的基準の設定が困難であることを示しています．

接尾辞（suffix）と後部連結形（FCF：final combining form）の区別：

多くの英語辞書が連結形と接辞を区別しており，連結形は語頭に位置する前部連結形と語末に位置する後部連結形に分類されます．しかし，筆者が目にした医学用語学習書の多くが連結形と呼んでいるのは前部連結形（ICF）に限られており，後部連結形に関する記述がありません．語末要素，つまり，後部連結形（FCF）と接尾辞（suffix）の両方を一括して接尾辞と定義している場合が多いようです．この方式は説明上の便利さはあるものの，接辞の定義上の問題にかかわるため（接頭辞と接尾辞は通常，直接結びつくことはないが，後部連結形を接尾辞と分類することにより接頭辞と接尾辞が直接連結する例ができてしまう．例，hyperpnea（過呼吸）：hyper-（prefix, 過度の）+ -pnea（FCF, 呼吸））．本書においては後部連結形と接尾辞を区別し，多くの辞書での分類上の定義に沿った方針を採用しています．皆さんが，ある程度詳しい英和辞典を利用する場合，語末要素は接尾辞と後部連結形に区分されていることが多いと思われますが，一般の医学用語学習書よりも詳しい定義を採用していることを念頭に置いてください．

2.3　連結母音（combining vowel）-o- / -i-

　前部連結形（ICF）の gastr- と後部連結形（FCF）の -tomy をつなぐ連結母音の -o- は本来，ギリシャ語系の要素を結合する際に用いられた母音ですが，fibroma「線維腫」のようにラテン語系の fibr(o)-「繊維・線維」とギリシャ語系の -oma「腫瘍」を連結しているような混血の例もみられます．医学用語において用いられる連結母音のほとんどは -o- ですが，ラテン語連結母音 -i- が用いられる場合は，ラテン語由来の複合語です（例，dorsiflexion「背屈」: dorsi-「背」ラテン語 *dorsum* より）．本来，ラテン語の連結母音は -i- が用いられていましたが，ギリシャ語系語彙がラテン語へ取り入れられ同化するに伴い，ギリシャ語で用いられていた -o- がラテン語の要素間（例，dorsolateral「背部側部の」），あるいは，ギリシャ語とラテン語の要素間の連結においても用いられるようになり（例，mammography「乳房造影」: mamm(o)-「乳房」＜ラテン語 *mamma*，-graphy「記録法，写法」＜ギリシャ語 *graphia*），今日では連結母音 -o- が広く用いられています．なお，連結母音 -o- は通常，前部連結形に付加されているものとして扱われることが多く，辞書や用語集では gastr(o)- や gastr/o- のような形式で提示されています．

　この連結母音 -o- は前部連結形が結びつく語末要素が子音の場合に現れ（例，図 1 の gastrotomy 参照），母音の場合に省かれます（例，図 2 の gastrectomy 参照）．ただし，医学用語によっては 2 つ以上の前部連結形を含んでいる場合があります．この場合，後ろの前部連結形が母音で始まっていても先頭の前部連結形には連結母音 -o- が現れます（図 5）．

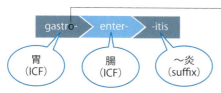

2 つの前部連結形（ICF）を含む場合の連結母音 -o-
後続の前部連結形 enter(o)- は母音で始まるが，gastr(o)- の連結母音は必要．一方，語末要素の接尾辞 -itis と連結される enter(o)- については連結母音 -o- は不要となる．

図 5　gastroenteritis（胃腸炎）の構造

　これまでの説明のポイントをまとめると次のようになります．
(1) 医学用語は接辞（affix）と連結形（combining form）から成立しており，どちらもほかの語や要素と結びついて用いられる．
(2) 接辞には接頭辞（prefix）と接尾辞（suffix）がある．
(3) 連結形には前部連結形（ICF）と後部連結形（FCF）がある．
(4) 前部連結形の連結母音（combining vowel）-o- は連結する相手となる語末要素が子音で始まる場合に現れる（ラテン語系においては連結母音として -i- が用いられる場合もある）．
(5) 接頭辞は連結母音なしにほかの語や連結形に直接結びつくことができる．
(6) 前部連結形（ICF）を 2 つ含む語の場合，2 つ目の前部連結形が母音で始まっていても 1 つ目の前部連結形には連結母音 -o- が現れる（図 5）．一方で語末要素（接尾辞と後部連結形（FCF））に直接連結する 2 つ目の前部連結形については，語末要素が母音で始まれば連結母音 -o- は現れない．
(7) 接辞や連結形はギリシャ語由来のもの，ラテン語由来のもの，同系統どうしを連結して用語をつくるのが原則であるが，この原則にあてはまらない例も存在する．

以上のまとめを念頭に置いて，医学用語の学習を進めてみましょう．基本的な接辞や連結形がある程度まで理解できれば，初出の医学用語であっても意味が類推できるようになります．図6をみてみましょう．接辞と連結形が規則どおりに結びつき，さまざまな医学用語をつくり出している統一感に筆者は美しさを感じますが，いかがでしょうか．今後の学習次第で，この図は無限に拡張することができます．新しい医学用語に出合うたびに，意味を類推し，確認しながら図6のような医学用語のネットワークを頭の中に広げていきましょう．

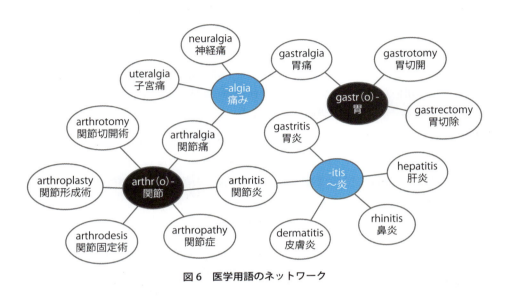

図6　医学用語のネットワーク

では，練習問題に解答してみましょう．

これまでの説明を読み返しつつ，巻末にある表1〜3や辞書，あるいはインターネット上のホームページ等を活用しながら解答しても結構です．練習問題を解きながら，医学用語の知識が自然と身につくはずです．

第Ⅱ部 医学用語の学習 123

練習問題

問題1 巻末リスト（表1〜3）を参考に，以下のフローチャートの空欄を埋めましょう．

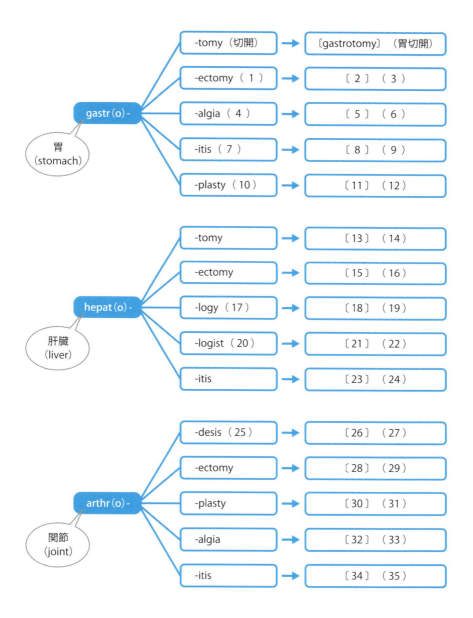

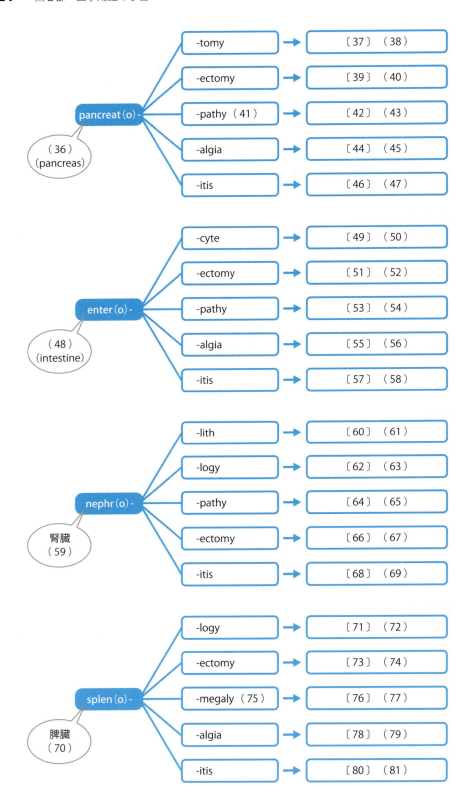

第Ⅱ部　医学用語の学習

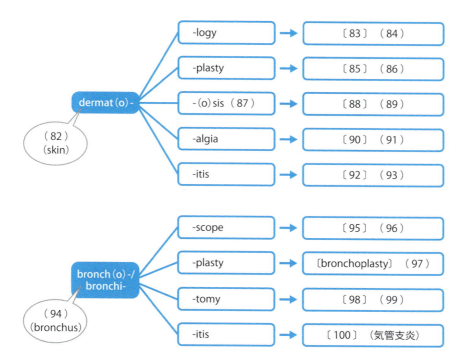

問題2　右枠内の接辞と連結形を用いて，空欄〔1〕〜〔60〕に適する用語を書きなさい．

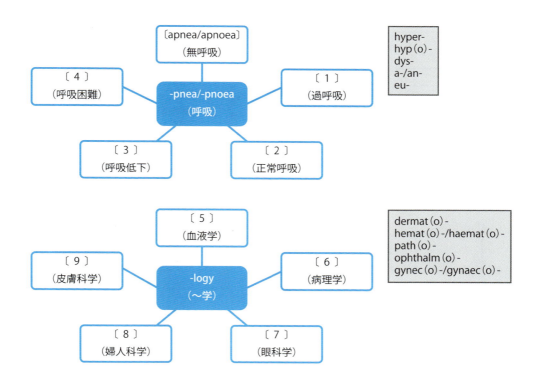

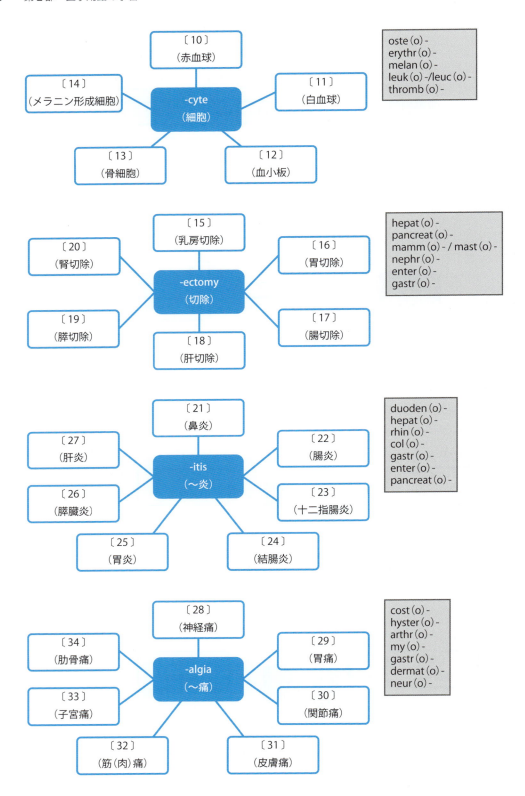

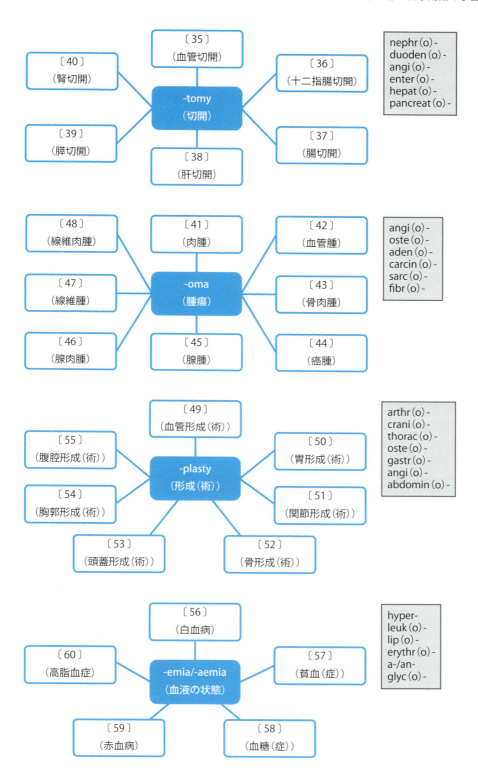

問題 3 次の各語を接辞や連結形に 3 分割し，日本語の意味を考えてみましょう．

(1) osteoarthritis（意味：変形性関節症/骨関節炎）*

(　　　　　)(　　　　　)(　　　　　)

*この病名に関して，現在は「変形性関節症」が広く用いられるため，英語の和訳とは一致しない．文字どおり訳すと「骨関節炎」となる．

(2) gastroenterology（意味：　　　　　）

(　　　　　)(　　　　　)(　　　　　)

(3) duodenoenterostomy（意味：　　　　　）

(　　　　　)(　　　　　)(　　　　　)

(4) pylorogastrectomy（意味：　　　　　）

(　　　　　)(　　　　　)(　　　　　)

(5) periodontitis（意味：　　　　　）

(　　　　　)(　　　　　)(　　　　　)

問題 4 次の各パーツを組み合わせてできるだけ多くの医学用語をつくってみましょう．

oste(o)-	carcin(o)-	-rrhage
hem(o)-	path(o)-	-oma
tetra-	hemi-	-gen
quadri-	sarc(o)-	-plegia

問題 5 次の（1）〜（5）の意味になるように単語のパーツを組み合わせてみましょう．必要なパーツは何回使用してもかまいません．

(1) 筋骨格系 　　〔　　1　　〕 system
(2) 心臓血管系 　〔　　2　　〕 system
(3) 脳血管系 　　〔　　3　　〕 system
(4) 心肺停止 　　〔　　4　　〕 arrest
(5) 脳脊髄液 　　〔　　5　　〕 fluid

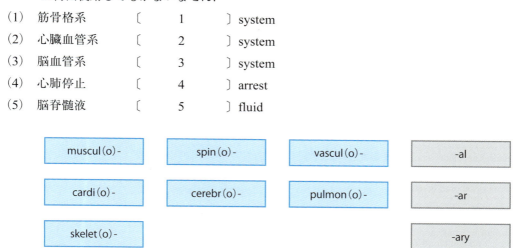

問題 6 巻末のリストや辞書を参考にしながら，下の図に新たな医学用語を書き加え，線でつないで図を拡張してみましょう．また，完成した図をお互いに発表してみましょう．

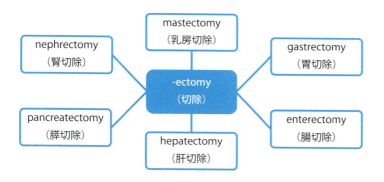

問題7 英語の定義を読んで，英語と日本語で適する医学用語を書きましょう．

No.	Definition(定義)	Medical Term(医学用語)	日本語
1	a medical condition causing painful inflammation and stiffness of the joints		
2	a substance that can cause cancer		
3	a specialist in the study and treatment of diseases of the heart		
4	the treatment of disease using chemicals, especially the treatment of cancer by cytotoxic drugs		
5	surgical removal of all or a portion of the colon		
6	a medical speciality concerned with the skin and its disorders		
7	difficult or labored breathing		
8	a red blood cell; a cell that carries oxygen from the lungs to the body tissues		
9	the scientific study and treatment of diseases of the blood and blood-forming organs		
10	a disease characterized by inflammation of the liver		
11	cancer of blood-forming tissues characterized by increased numbers of abnormal leukocytes		
12	inflammation of the duodenum		
13	a medical speciality concerned with the study and treatment of diseases of the eye		
14	X-ray examination of the breasts to diagnose and locate tumors		
15	pain in the stomach		
16	inflammation of the mucous membrane of the nose		
17	a microorganism such as a bacterium or a virus which can cause disease		
18	a doctor's opinion about the likely course of a medical condition		
19	a medical speciality dealing with the reproductive system of women and its diseases		
20	a profuse discharge of blood from ruptured blood vessels		
21	an illness that causes an abnormally fast passage of waste material through the large intestine in liquid rather than solid form		
22	paralysis of one side of the body as the result of disease of or injury to the motor centers of the brain		
23	abnormally rapid or deep breathing		
24	a medical speciality dealing with the correction of deformities of bones or muscles		
25	an instrument using a fiber-optic technology to visualize the internal parts of the body for diagnostic or therapeutic purposes		
26	the spread of cancer cells from their initial site in the body to another part of the body		
27	extreme or irrational fear of being in a high place		
28	a gene having the potential to transform a normal cell into a cancerous cell		

(前ページのつづき)

No.	Definition（定義）	Medical Term（医学用語）	日本語
29	a chronic disorder characterized by excessive drinking of alcohol leading to psychological and physical dependence or addiction		
30	inflammation of the womb		
31	relating to the heart and blood vessels		
32	surgical removal of all or a portion of the stomach		
33	an outbreak of a disease that affects an exceptionally high proportion of the population over a wide area		
34	a substance that can destroy bacteria		
35	an instrument for the precise measurement of angles		
36	a medical speciality concerned with children and their diseases		
37	the identification of diseases by the examination of symptoms		
38	the study and treatment of mental disorders		
39	a surgical incision into the larynx		
40	a slightly bluish color of the skin caused by a deficiency of oxygen in the blood		
41	relating to the brain and spinal cord		
42	relating to or occurring after a medical operation		
43	paralysis of all four extremities		
44	surgical removal of the pancreas		
45	relating to both musculature and skeleton		
46	inflammation of the oesophagus		
47	the start of cancer formation		
48	a temporary inability to breathe		
49	relating to the heart and lungs		
50	surgical removal of one or both ovaries		

参考文献

1) Bauer, L. (1983). English Word-formation. Cambridge: Cambridge University Press.
2) Chabner, D-E. (2012). Medical Terminology A Short Course, Sixth Edition. St. Louis: Saunders.
3) Cohen, B. J. (2011). Medical Terminology An Illustrated Guide, Sixth Edition. Philadelphia: Lippincott Williams & Wilkins.
4) Fremgen, B. F. & Frucht, S. S. (2013). Medical Terminology A Living Language, Fifth Edition. New Jersey: Pearson Education, Inc.
5) Huddleston, R. & Pullum, G. K. (2002). The Cambridge Grammar of the English Language. Cambridge: Cambridge University Press.
6) Hutton, A. R. (2006). An Introduction to Medical Terminology for Health Care, Fourth Edition. London: Churchill Livingstone.
7) 家入葉子（2007）.『ベーシック英語史』東京：ひつじ書房.
8) 児馬　修（1996）.『ファンダメンタル英語史』東京：ひつじ書房.
9) 中島文雄（1979）.『英語発達史　改訂版』東京：岩波書店.
10) 中尾俊夫，寺島廸子（1988）.『図説　英語史入門』東京：大修館書店.
11) 西川盛雄（2006）.『英語接辞研究』東京：開拓社.
12) 大塚高信・中島文雄（1982）.『新英語学辞典』東京：研究社.
13) 寺澤　盾（2008）.『英語の歴史　過去から未来への物語』東京：中央公論社.
14) Turley, S. (2011). Medical Language, Second Edition. New Jersey: Pearson Education, Inc.
15) 梅田　修（1990）.『英語の語源事典』東京：大修館書店.

参照辞書

1) Cambridge Advanced Learner's Dictionary, Third Edition (2008). Cambridge: Cambridge University Press.
2) Collins English Dictionary, Eleventh Edition (2011). Glasgow: HarperCollins Publishers.
3) ジーニアス英和大辞典（2001）．東京：大修館書店.
4) Longman Dictionary of Contemporary English, Fifth Edition (2009). Essex: Pearson Education Limited.
5) Macmillan English Dictionary for Advanced Learners, Second Edition (2007). Oxford: Macmillan Education.
6) Oxford Dictionary of English, Third Edition (2010). Oxford: Oxford University Press.
7) ランダムハウス英和大辞典，第2版（1993）．東京：小学館.
8) リーダーズ英和辞典，第2版（1999）．東京：研究社.
9) リーダーズ・プラス（2000）．東京：研究社.
10) 新英和大辞典，第6版（2002）．東京：研究社.
11) 新和英大辞典，第5版　電子増補版（2003）．東京：研究社.
12) Shorter Oxford English Dictionary on Historical Principles, Sixth Edition (2007). Oxford: Oxford

University Press.
13) ステッドマン医学大辞典，改訂第6版（英和・和英）（2008）．東京：メジカルビュー社．
14) The Oxford English Dictionary, Second Edition（1991）. Oxford: Oxford University Press.
15) Webster's Third New International Dictionary of the English Language Unabridged（2002）. Massachusetts: Merriam-Webster Inc.

略号一覧（アルファベット順）
FCF：Final Combining Form（後部連結形）
G：Greek（ギリシャ語由来）
ICF：Initial Combining Form（前部連結形）
L：Latinate（ラテン語由来）
OE：Old English（古英語）
Pref.：Prefix（接頭辞）
Suf.：Suffix（接尾辞）

表1　医学用語─語頭要素・語末要素（接頭辞・前部連結形・接尾辞・後部連結形）アルファベット順一覧

	接辞と連結形	語源	接辞と連結形の分類	関連分野	意味（英語）	用例（日本語）	用例解説
1	a- / an-	G	Pref.	一般性が高い接頭辞	不・無・非 (not / without)	apnea（無呼吸）	-pnea / -pnoea「呼吸」
2	ab-	L	Pref.	一般性が高い接頭辞	〜から離れた (away from)	abnormal（異常な）	normal「標準の・正常の」
3	abdomin(o)-	L	ICF	体の部分	腹部（abdomen）	abdominal（腹部の）	-al 接尾辞「〜の」
4	-able	L	Suf.	一般性が高い接尾辞	〜できる（can）	curable（治療できる）	curabilis（ラテン語，= cure + -able）より
5	-acousia	G	FCF	医学・医療・学問	聴覚・聴取 (condition of hearing)	dysacousia（聴覚不全）	dys-「困難な」
6	acr(o)-	G	ICF	大小・形・色・数・量・状態・位置	先端・頂上 (top / peak / summit)	acrophobia（高所恐怖症）	-phobia「恐怖症」
7	acromi(o)-	L	ICF	筋・骨格系	肩峰（acromion）	acromioclavicular（肩峰鎖骨の）	clavicular「鎖骨の」
8	aden(o)-	G	ICF	体関連物質	腺（gland）	adenocarcinoma（腺癌）	carcinoma「癌腫」
9	aer(o)-	G	ICF	自然界の諸要素	空気（air）	aerophagia（空気嚥下）	-phagia / -phagy「食べること」
10	-agra	G	FCF	病気・症状	疼痛発作 (sudden pain)	podagra（足部痛風）	pod(o)-「足」
11	-al	L	Suf.	一般性が高い接尾辞	〜に関する・〜の (relating to)	esophageal（食道の）	esophag(o)-「食道」
12	albumin(o)-	L	ICF	体関連物質	蛋白（albumin）	albuminous（アルブミン・蛋白の）	-ous「〜を持つ・〜の特徴を有する」
13	alg(o)-	G	ICF	感覚器系	痛み（pain）	algometry（痛覚検査）	-metry「測定（法）」
14	-algia	G	FCF	病気・症状	〜痛（pain）	hepatalgia（肝臓痛）	hepat(o)-「肝臓」
15	alveol(o)-	L	ICF	呼吸器系	肺胞／歯槽（alveolus）	alveolitis（肺胞炎）	-itis「〜炎」
16	ana-	G	Pref.	一般性が高い接頭辞	上・後・再 (up / back / again)	analysis（分析）	-lysis「分解」
17	angi(o)-	G	ICF	心臓・血管・リンパ系	血管（blood vessel）	angioma（血管腫）	-oma「腫・瘤」
18	anis(o)-	G	ICF	大小・形・色・数・量・状態・位置	不等（unequal）	anisodactylous（不等指症の）	dactyl-「指・足指」
19	ante-	L	Pref.	一般性が高い接頭辞	前の（before）	antebrachial（前腕の）	brachial「腕の」（⇔ post-）
20	anti-	G	Pref.	一般性が高い接頭辞	反・対・抗 (against / preventing)	antibacterial（抗菌性の）	bacterial「細菌の」
21	aort(o)-	L	ICF	心臓・血管・リンパ系	大動脈（aorta）	aortitis（大動脈炎）	-itis「〜炎」
22	append(o)- / appendic(o)-	L	ICF	消化器系	虫垂（appendix）	appendectomy / appendicectomy（虫垂切除術）	-ectomy「切除（術）」
23	aqua- / aqui-	L	ICF	自然界の諸要素	水（water）	aqueous（水の・水溶性の・水を含む）	-eous 接尾辞「〜の性質を持つ」
24	arteri(o)-	G	ICF	心臓・血管・リンパ系	動脈（artery）	arteriosclerosis（動脈硬化症）	sclerosis「硬化症」
25	arthr(o)-	G	ICF	筋・骨格系	関節（joint）	arthritis（関節炎）	-itis「〜炎」
26	-ary	L	Suf.	一般性が高い接尾辞	〜に関する・〜の (pertaining to)	pulmonary（肺の）	pulmon(o)-「肺」
27	audi(o)-	L	ICF	感覚器系	聴覚（hearing），音（sound）	audiometry（聴力測定）	-metry「測定（法）」
28	aur(i)-	L	ICF	感覚器系	耳（ear）	aural（耳の）	-al 接尾辞「〜の」
29	aut(o)-	G	ICF	大小・形・色・数・量・状態・位置	自己（self），自動の（by itself）	autoantibody（自己抗体）	antibody「抗体」
30	bi-	L	ICF	大小・形・色・数・量・状態・位置	2（two / double）	bisexual（両性素質の）	sexual「性の」
31	bi(o)-	G	ICF	自然界の諸要素	生命（life）	biopsy（生検）	-opsy「見ること」⇒「検査」

（次ページに続く）

(表1のつづき)

	接辞と連結形	語源	接辞と連結形の分類	関連分野	意味(英語)	用例(日本語)	用例解説
32	-blast	G	FCF	医学・医療・学問	芽(sprout), 胚(embryo)	angioblast(血管芽細胞)	angi(o)-「血管」
33	blast(o)-	L	ICF	心臓・血管・リンパ系	胚(embryo), 芽(sprout / germ)	blastoma(芽腫)	-oma「腫・瘤」
34	brachi(o)-	L	ICF	体の部分	腕(arm), 上腕(upper arm)	brachialgia(上腕痛)	-algia「〜痛」
35	brady-	G	ICF	大小・形・色・数・量・状態・位置	遅い(slow)	bradykinesia(動作緩慢)	-kinesia「運動」
36	bronch(o)- / bronchi(o)-	G	ICF	呼吸器系	気管支(bronchus)	bronchoscope(気管支鏡)	-scope「見る器械」
37	carcin(o)-	G	ICF	病気・症状	癌(cancer)	carcinogen(発癌物質)	-gen「〜を生むもの」
38	cardi(o)-	G	ICF	心臓・血管・リンパ系	心臓(heart), 噴門(cardia)	cardiologist(心臓病専門医)	-logist「〜の研究者」
39	carp(o)-	G	ICF	筋・骨格系	手根(wrist)	radiocarpal(橈骨手根骨の)	radi(o)-「橈骨」
40	-cele	G	FCF	病気・症状	腫瘍・ヘルニア(tumor / hernia)	hematocele(血瘤)	hemat(o)-「血」
41	cent(i)-	L	ICF	大小・形・色・数・量・状態・位置	1/100(one hundredth)	centimeter / centimetre(センチメートル)	ギリシャ語系の数は整数、ラテン語系の数は分数を表す
42	cephal(o)-	G	ICF	体の部分	頭部(head)	cephalomegaly(頭部巨大症)	-megaly「(〜の部分の)巨大(症)」
43	-cephalus	G	FCF	病気・症状	頭部異常(abnormal condition of the head)	hydrocephalus(水頭症)	hydr(o)-「水」
44	cerat(o)- / kerat(o)-	G	ICF	感覚器系	角膜(cornea)	keratitis(角膜炎)	-itis「〜炎」
45	cerebell(o)- / cerebelli-	L	ICF	脳神経系	小脳(cerebellum)	cerebellar(小脳の)	-ar 接尾辞「〜の」
46	cerebr(o)-	L	ICF	脳神経系	脳(brain), 大脳(cerebrum)	cerebrospinal(脳脊髄の)	spinal「背骨の・脊髄の」
47	cervic(o)-	L	ICF	体の部分	首・頸部(neck / cervix)	cervicography(子宮頸管撮影)	-graphy「写法」
48	cheil(o)- / chil(o)-	G	ICF	消化器系	唇(lip)	cheilotomy(口唇切開術)	-tomy「切開(術)」
49	chem(o)-	L	ICF	医学・医療・学問	化学の(chemical)	chemotherapy(化学療法)	therapy「治療」
50	chlor(o)-	G	ICF	大小・形・色・数・量・状態・位置	緑(green)	chlorophyl(葉緑素)	-phyl(l)「植物内の〜色素」
51	chol(o)- / chole-	G	ICF	体関連物質	胆汁(bile / gall)	cholelith(胆石)	-lith「結石」
52	cholecyst(o)-	L	ICF	消化器系	胆嚢(gallbladder / cholecyst)	cholecystitis(胆嚢炎)	-itis「〜炎」
53	chondr(o)- / chondri-	G	ICF	筋・骨格系	軟骨(cartilage)	chondrocyte(軟骨細胞)	-cyte「細胞」
54	chrom(o)- / chromat(o)-	G	ICF	大小・形・色・数・量・状態・位置	色(color)	chromatopsia(色視症:物が異常に着色されてみえる状態)	-opsia「〜視」
55	-cide	L	FCF	医学・医療・学問	〜を殺す薬剤(agent that kills)	bactericide(殺菌剤)	bacteri-「細菌」
56	circum-	L	Pref.	一般性が高い接頭辞	周囲に・取り巻く(around)	circumoral(口腔周囲の)	oral「口(腔)の」
57	-clasis	G	FCF	病気・症状	崩壊(breaking)	erythroclasis(赤血球崩壊)	erythr(o)-「赤・赤血球」
58	clavi- / clav(o)-	L	ICF	筋・骨格系	鎖骨(clavicle)	clavipectoral fascia(鎖骨胸筋筋膜)	pectoral「胸筋の」, fascia「筋膜」
59	-cle / -cule	L	Suf.	一般性が高い接尾辞	小〜(small)	saccule(小嚢)	ラテン語系名詞接尾辞
60	co-	L	Pref.	一般性が高い接頭辞	共同の・相互の・副(jointly / mutually)	cocarcinogen(発癌補助物質)	carcinogen「発癌物質」
61	col(o)-	G	ICF	消化器系	結腸(colon)	colectomy(結腸切除)	-ectomy「切除(術)」

(次ページに続く)

(表1のつづき)

	接辞と連結形	語源	接辞と連結形の分類	関連分野	意味（英語）	用例（日本語）	用例解説
62	colp(o)-	G	ICF	生殖器系	腟(vagina)	colpitis(腟炎)(= vaginitis)	-itis「～炎」
63	contra-	L	Pref.	一般性が高い接頭辞	反対・逆(against / opposite)	contraception(避妊)	contra- + (con)ception「妊娠・受胎」
64	cortic(o)-	L	ICF	体の部分	(大脳／副腎)皮質(cortex)	corticosteroid(コルチコステロイド)	steroid「ステロイド」
65	cost(o)-	L	ICF	筋・骨格系	肋骨(rib)	costectomy(肋骨切除)	-ectomy「切除（術）」
66	crani(o)-	G	ICF	筋・骨格系	頭蓋骨(cranium)	craniometry(頭蓋骨計測法)	-metry「測定法」
67	crypt(o)-	G	ICF	一般性が高い接頭辞	隠された(hidden)	cryptogenic(原因不明の)	-genic「～を生み出す・遺伝子を有する」
68	cyan(o)-	G	ICF	大小・形・色・数・量・状態・位置	藍(dark blue)	cyanosis(チアノーゼ)	-osis「病的状態」
69	cyst(o)-	G	ICF	泌尿器系	膀胱(urinary bladder)	cystolith(膀胱結石)	-lith「結石」
70	cyt(o)-	G	ICF	体関連物質	細胞(cell)	cytoplasm(細胞質)	-plasm「形成するもの」
71	-cyte	G	FCF	医学・医療・学問	細胞(cell)	erythrocyte(赤血球)	erythr(o)-「赤・赤血球」
72	dactyl(o)-	G	ICF	体の部分	指(finger)	dactyloscopy(指紋検査)	-scopy「検査・観察」
73	de-	L	Pref.	一般性が高い接頭辞	分離(away), 下降(down from)	deform(～の形を損なう)	form「形づくる」
74	dec(a)-	G	ICF	大小・形・色・数・量・状態・位置	10(ten)	decagon(十角形)	-gon「～角形」
75	deci-	L	ICF	大小・形・色・数・量・状態・位置	10分の1(one tenth)	deciliter / decilitre(デシリットル)	liter / litre「リットル（容量の単位）」
76	dem(o)-	G	ICF	人間一般	人々(people)	demography(人口統計学)	-graphy「記述法」
77	dent(o)- / denti-	L	ICF	消化器系	歯(tooth)	dental(歯の)	-al 接尾辞「～の」
78	-derma	G	FCF	医学・医療・学問	皮膚(skin)	scleroderma(硬皮症)	scler(o)-「堅い」
79	dermat(o)- / derma- / derm(o)-	G	ICF	感覚器官	皮膚(skin)	dermatology(皮膚科学)	-logy「学問」
80	-desis	G	FCF	医学・医療・学問	束縛・接合(binding together by surgery)	arthrodesis(関節固定(術))	arthr(o)-「関節」
81	dextr(o)-	L	ICF	大小・形・色・数・量・状態・位置	右(right)	dextrocardia(右胸心)	-cardia「心臓の働き・位置」
82	di-	G	Pref.	一般性が高い接頭辞	2(two / twice / double)	dioxide(二酸化物)	oxide「酸化物」
83	dia-	G	Pref.	一般性が高い接頭辞	通して・横切って・離れて(through / across / apart)	diagnosis(診断)	-gnosis「認識」
84	dipl(o)-	G	ICF	大小・形・色・数・量・状態・位置	2(two / double)	diplococcus(双球菌)	coccus「球菌」
85	dis-	L	Pref.	一般性が高い接頭辞	不・無・非(not / opposite of / absence of)	disability(障害，無能)	ability「能力」
86	dist(o)-	L	ICF	大小・形・色・数・量・状態・位置	末端の・遠位の(distal)	distal(遠位の)	-al 接尾辞「～の」
87	dors(o)- / dorsi-	L	ICF	体の部分	背(back)	dorsolateral(背部側部の)	lateral「側面の」
88	-drome	G	FCF	医学・医療・学問	競走路(course), 走る(running)	syndrome(症候群)	syn-「同時に」
89	duoden(o)-	L	ICF	消化器系	十二指腸(duodenum)	duodenal ulcer(十二指腸潰瘍)	-al 接尾辞「～の」
90	dys-	G	ICF	大小・形・色・数・量・状態・位置	悪化(bad), 困難な(difficult)	dyspnea(呼吸困難)	-pnea / -pnoea「呼吸」
91	eco-	G	ICF	自然界の諸要素	生態(学)(ecology)	ecosystem(生態系)	system「系」

(次ページに続く)

(表1のつづき)

	接辞と連結形	語源	接辞と連結形の分類	関連分野	意味（英語）	用例（日本語）	用例解説
92	ect(o)-	G	ICF	大小・形・色・数・量・状態・位置	外の (external)	ectocornea（角膜上皮）	cornea「角膜」
93	-ectomy	G	FCF	医学・医療・学問	切除（術）(excision)	gastrectomy（胃切除（術））	gastr(o)-「胃」
94	electr(o)-	G	ICF	医学・医療・学問	電気 (electricity)	electrocardiography（心電図検査）	cardiography「心拍記録(法)」
95	em-	L	Pref.	一般性が高い接頭辞	中に入れる (put into), 〜の状態にす (bring into the condition of)	embalm（死体に防腐処置をする）	balm「芳香性樹脂」
96	-emia / -aemia / -hemia / -haemia	G	FCF	病気・症状	〜な血液を有する状態 (blood condition)	leukemia / leukaemia（白血病）	leuk(o)- / leuc(o)-「白・白血球」
97	en-	L	Pref.	一般性が高い接頭辞	中に入れる (put into), 〜の状態にする (bring into the condition of)	enrich（富ませる）	rich「金持ちの・豊かな」
98	encephal(o)-	G	ICF	脳神経系	脳 (brain)	encephalocele（脳ヘルニア）	-cele「ヘルニア」
99	end(o)-	G	ICF	大小・形・色・数・量・状態・位置	内部 (within)	endoscopy（内視鏡検査）	-scopy「検査・観察」
100	ennea-	G	ICF	大小・形・色・数・量・状態・位置	9 (nine)	enneagon（九角形）	-gon「〜角形」
101	enter(o)-	G	ICF	消化器系	腸 (intestine)	enterobacteria（腸内細菌）	bacteria「細菌 (bacterium)」の複数形
102	epi-	G	Pref.	一般性が高い接頭辞	上 (upon / above)	epidemic（流行性の / 流行(病)）	epi- + demos「人々（ギリシャ語）」+ -ic「〜の: 接尾辞」cf. pandemic
103	episio-	G	ICF	生殖器系	外陰 (vulva)	episiotomy（会陰切開（術））	-tomy「〜切開（術）」
104	equi-	L	ICF	大小・形・色・数・量・状態・位置	等しい (equal)	equicaloric（等カロリーの）	caloric「カロリーの」
105	-er	OE	Suf.	一般性が高い接尾辞	〜する人(もの) (a person or thing that performs the action described by the verb)	helper（助手）	help「助ける」
106	erythr(o)-	G	ICF	大小・形・色・数・量・状態・位置	赤 (red), 赤血球 (erythrocyte)	erythrocyte（赤血球）	-cyte「細胞」cf. leukocyte（白血球）, thrombocyte（血小板）
107	esophag(o)- / oesophag(o)-	G	ICF	消化器系	食道 (esophagus / oesophagus)	esophagitis / oesophagitis（食道炎）	-itis「〜炎」
108	eu-	G	ICF	大小・形・色・数・量・状態・位置	良 (well / good)	eupnea（正常呼吸）	-pnea / -pnoea「呼吸」
109	ex-	G	Pref.	一般性が高い接頭辞	外に (out)	excrete（排出する・分泌する）	excrenere「排出する（ラテン語）」より, ex-「外へ」+ cerenere「篩にかける・より分ける」
110	exo-	G	Pref.	一般性が高い接頭辞	外 (external / from outside)	exocrine（外分泌(性)の）	exo- + crine「分離する（ギリシャ語）」(⇔ endocrine)
111	extra-	L	Pref.	一般性が高い接頭辞	〜外の (outside / beyond)	extracarpal（手根外の）	carpal「手根(骨)の」
112	fibr(o)-	L	ICF	体関連物質	線維 (fiber)	fibroadenoma（線維腺腫）	adenoma「腺腫」
113	fore-	OE	ICF	大小・形・色・数・量・状態・位置	前の (the front part of / before)	forearm（前腕）, forehead（額）	arm「腕」, head「頭」
114	gangli(o)-	G	ICF	脳神経系	神経節 (ganglion)	ganglioma（神経節腫）	-oma「腫・瘤」
115	gastr(o)-	G	ICF	消化器系	胃 (stomach)	gastralgia（胃痛）	-algia「〜痛」
116	-gen	G	FCF	医学・医療・学問	〜を生じるもの (a substance that produces something)	pathogen（病原菌, 病原体）	path(o)-「病気, 苦痛」

（次ページに続く）

(表1のつづき)

	接辞と連結形	語源	接辞と連結形の分類	関連分野	意味（英語）	用例（日本語）	用例解説
117	-genesis	G	FCF	医学・医療・学問	発生・形成 (formation)	carcinogenesis（発癌）	carcin(o)-「癌」
118	-genic	G	FCF	医学・医療・学問	〜を生み出す (producing)	carcinogenic（発癌性の）	carcin(o)-「癌」
119	-genous	G	FCF	医学・医療・学問	〜を生み出す (producing)、〜によって発生する (originating in)	myelogenous（骨髄性の）	myel(o)-「骨髄・脊髄」
120	geront(o)-	G	ICF	大小・形・色・数・量・状態・位置	老人 (old man)、老齢 (old age)	gerontology（老人学・老年学）	-logy「学問」
121	gingiv(o)-	L	ICF	消化器系	歯肉 (gum)	gingivitis（歯肉炎）	-itis「〜炎」
122	glauc(o)-	G	ICF	大小・形・色・数・量・状態・位置	緑灰色の (bluish-grey)	glaucoma（緑内障）	*glaukoma*「水晶体の濁り」（ギリシャ語）より
123	gloss(o)-	L	ICF	消化器系	舌 (tongue)	glossoplegia（舌麻痺）	-plegia「麻痺」
124	glyc(o)- / gluc(o)-	G	ICF	体関連物質	糖 (sugar)	glycogen（グリコーゲン）	-gen「〜を生じるもの」
125	-gnosia	G	FCF	医学・医療・学問	認識 (recognition)	agnosia（失認）	a- / an-「不・無・非」
126	-gnosis	G	FCF	医学・医療・学問	認識 (recognition)	prognosis（予後）	pro-「前」
127	-gram	G	FCF	医学・医療・学問	記録 (record)	electrocardiogram（心電図）	electr(o)-「電気」, cardi(o)-「心臓」
128	-graph	G	FCF	医学・医療・学問	記録計器 (instrument for recording)	electrocardiograph（心電計）	electr(o)-「電気」, cardi(o)-「心臓」
129	-graphy	G	FCF	医学・医療・学問	写法・記録法 (process of recording)	electrocardiography（心電図記録法）	electr(o)-「電気」, cardi(o)-「心臓」
130	gynec(o)- / gynaec(o)-	G	ICF	自然界の諸要素	女性 (woman)	gynecology / gynaecology（婦人科学）	-logy「学問」
131	hect(o)-	G	ICF	大小・形・色・数・量・状態・位置	100 (hundred)	hectare（ヘクタール：100アールに相当）	ギリシャ語系の数は整数、ラテン語系の数は分数を表す
132	hemat(o)- / haemat(o)- / hem(o)- / haem(o)- / hema- / haema-	G	ICF	心臓・血管・リンパ系	血液 (blood)	hematology（血液学）	-logy「学問」
133	hemi-	G	ICF	大小・形・色・数・量・状態・位置	半分 (half)	hemiplegia（半側麻痺）	-plegia「麻痺」
134	hepat(o)-	G	ICF	消化器系	肝臓 (liver)	hepatitis（肝炎）	-itis「〜炎」
135	hept(a)-	G	ICF	大小・形・色・数・量・状態・位置	7 (seven)	heptahedron（七面体）	-hedron「〜面体」
136	heter(o)-	G	ICF	大小・形・色・数・量・状態・位置	異 (different)	heterogenous（外来の、外生の）	-genous「〜によって発生する・〜を生じる」
137	hex(a)-	G	ICF	大小・形・色・数・量・状態・位置	6 (six)	hexahedron（六面体）	-hedron「〜面体」
138	hidr(o)-	G	ICF	体関連物質	汗 (sweat)	hidrosis（過剰発汗）	-osis「病的状態」
139	hom(o)-	G	ICF	大小・形・色・数・量・状態・位置	同 (same)	homosexual（同性愛の）	sexual「性の」
140	humer(o)-	L	ICF	筋・骨格系	上腕(骨) (humerus) の	humeral（上腕骨の）	-al 接尾辞「〜の」
141	hydr(o)-	G	ICF	自然界の諸要素	水 (water)	hydrocephalus（水頭症）	-cephalus「頭部異常」
142	hyp(o)-	G	Pref.	一般性が高い接頭辞	下の・不足の (below / deficient)	hypoacidity（低酸症）	acidity「酸(性)度」（⇔ hyper-）
143	hyper-	G	Pref.	一般性が高い接頭辞	過度の (over / excessive)	hyperpnea（過呼吸）	-pnea / -pnoea「呼吸」
144	hyster(o)-	G	ICF	生殖器系	子宮 (uterus / womb)	hysterotomy（子宮切開）	-tomy「切開(術)」

（次ページに続く）

(表1のつづき)

	接辞と連結形	語源	接辞と連結形の分類	関連分野	意味（英語）	用例（日本語）	用例解説
145	-ia	G	FCF	病気・症状	病名をつくる (forming names of disorders)	leukemia / leukaemia（白血病）	ギリシャ語・ラテン語系名詞接尾辞
146	-iasis	G	Suf.	病気・症状	〜性の病気 (forming names of disorders)	psoriasis（乾癬）	*psora*「かゆみ（ギリシャ語）」
147	-iatrics	G	FCF	医学・医療・学問	医療・治療 (medical treatment)	pediatrics / paediatrics（小児科学）	ped(o)- / paed(o)-「子供」
148	-iatry	G	FCF	医学・医療・学問	医療・治療 (medical treatment)	psychiatry（精神医学）	psych(o)-「精神」
149	-ician	F	Suf.	一般性が高い接尾辞	〜の専門家 (specialist)	pediatrician（小児科医）	pediatric「小児科の」
150	-ics	G	Suf.	医学・医療・学問	〜学(science), 〜術(art)	orthopaedics / orthopedics（整形外科学）	orth(o)-「正しい」, p(a)ed(o)-「子供」
151	-iform / -form	L	FCF	大小・形・色・数・量・状態・位置	〜の形を持つ (having the form of)	cuneiform（楔状骨の）	*cuneus*「楔（ラテン語）」
152	il-	L	Pref.	一般性が高い接頭辞	不・無・非(not)	illegal（違法の）	legal（適法の）
153	ile(o)-	L	ICF	消化器系	回腸(ileum)	ileocolitis（回結腸炎）	-col(o)「結腸」, -itis「〜炎」
154	ili(o)-	L	ICF	筋・骨格系	腸骨(ilium)	iliofemoral（腸骨と大腿骨の）	femoral「大腿骨の」
155	im-	L	Pref.	一般性が高い接頭辞	不・無・非(not)	impossible（不可能な）	possible「可能な」
156	immun(o)-	L	ICF	人間一般	免疫(immunity)	immunodeficiency（免疫不全）	deficiency「欠乏・不足」
157	in-[1]	L	Pref.	一般性が高い接頭辞	中へ(into)	include（含む）	*includere*「囲む・閉じ込める（ラテン語）」より，in- + *claudere*「閉じる」
158	in-[2]	L	Pref.	一般性が高い接頭辞	不・無・非(not)	infertility（生殖不能）	fertility「受胎能力」
159	infra-	L	Pref.	一般性が高い接頭辞	下に・〜の下の (below)	infraclavicular（鎖骨下の）	clavicular「鎖骨(clavicle)の」
160	inter-	L	Pref.	一般性が高い接頭辞	間・相互の (between / among)	intervertebral（脊椎間の）	vertebral「脊椎の」
161	intra-	L	Pref.	一般性が高い接頭辞	内の(within / inside)	intravascular（血管内の）	vascular「血管の」
162	intro-	L	Pref.	一般性が高い接頭辞	中に(to the inside)	introvert（内向性の）	*introvetere*（ラテン語，intro- + *vertere*「回転する・向く」）
163	ir-	L	Pref.	一般性が高い接頭辞	不・無・非(not)	irregular（不規則な）	regular（規則的な）
164	is(o)-	G	ICF	大小・形・色・数・量・状態・位置	等(equal)	isogenic（同質遺伝子型の）	-genic「遺伝子の」
165	ischi(o)-	G	ICF	筋・骨格系	坐骨(ischium)	ischial（坐骨の）	-al 接尾辞「〜の」
166	-ism	G	Suf.	病気・症状	病的状態 (abnormal condition)	alcoholism（アルコール依存症）	alcohol「アルコール」
167	-ist	G	Suf.	一般性が高い接尾辞	〜の専門家 (specialist)	orthopaedist / orthopedist（整形外科医）	orth(o)-「正しい」, p(a)ed(o)-「子供」
168	-istic	G	Suf.	一般性が高い接尾辞	〜に関する・〜の (relating to)	linguistic（言語の）	lingu(o)-「言語・舌」
169	-itis	G	Suf.	病気・症状	〜炎(inflammation)	dermatitis（皮膚炎）	dermat(o)-「皮膚」
170	-ize / -ise	G	Suf.	一般性が高い接尾辞	〜化する (make / become)	minimize（最小にする）	minim(um)「最低限度」+ -ize
171	jejun(o)-	L	ICF	消化器系	空腸(jejunum)	jejunostomy（空腸造瘻術）	-stomy「開口術」
172	kerat(o)- / cerat(o)-	G	ICF	感覚器系	角膜(cornea)	keratitis（角膜炎）	-itis「〜炎」
173	kil(o)-	G	ICF	大小・形・色・数・量・状態・位置	1000(thousand)	kilogram（キログラム）	ギリシャ語系の数は整数，ラテン語系の数は分数を表す

(次ページに続く)

(表1のつづき)

	接辞と連結形	語源	接辞と連結形の分類	関連分野	意味（英語）	用例（日本語）	用例解説
174	kinesi(o)-	G	ICF	大小・形・色・数・量・状態・位置	動き (movement)	kinesitherapy / kinesiotherapy（運動療法）	therapy「治療・療法」
175	-kinesia	G	FCF	医学・医療・学問	運動 (movement), 筋運動 (muscular activity)	bradykinesia（動作緩慢）	brady-「遅い・緩慢な」
176	-kinesis	G	FCF	医学・医療・学問	運動 (movement, activity)	chemokinesis（化学運動性）	chem(o)-「化学の」
177	labi(o)-	L	ICF	消化器系	唇 (lip)	labiodental（唇歯音の）	dental「歯音の」
178	lact(o)-	L	ICF	体関連物質	乳 (milk)	lactoprotein（乳蛋白質）	protein「蛋白」
179	lapar(o)-	G	ICF	体の部分	脇腹 (flank), 腹壁 (abdominal wall)	laparoscope（腹腔鏡）	-scope「見る器械」
180	laryng(o)-	G	ICF	呼吸器系	喉頭 (larynx)	laryngotomy（喉頭切開）	-tomy「切開（術）」
181	laryng(o)-	G	ICF	体の部分	喉頭 (larynx)	laryngotomy（喉頭切開）	-tomy「切開（術）」
182	leuc(o)- / leuk(o)-	G	ICF	心臓・血管・リンパ系	白 (white), 白血球 (leucocyte / leukocyte)	leukemia / leukaemia（白血病）	-emia / -aemia「血液の状態」 cf. erythrocyte, thrombocyte
183	leuc(o)- / leuk(o)-	G	ICF	大小・形・色・数・量・状態・位置	白 (white), 白血球 (leucocyte / leukocyte)	leukemia / leukaemia（白血病）	-emia / -aemia「血液の状態」 cf. erythrocyte, thrombocyte
184	-lexia	G	FCF	病気・症状	〜な（欠陥のある）読み方 (condition of speech)	dyslexia（難読症）	dys-「困難な」
185	lingu(o)- / lingui-	L	ICF	人間一般	言語 (language), 舌 (tongue)	linguistic（言語の）	-istic 形容詞をつくる接尾辞「〜の」
186	lip(o)-	G	ICF	体関連物質	脂肪 (fat)	lipocyte（脂肪細胞）	-cyte「細胞」
187	-lith	G	Suf.	病気・症状	石・結石 (stone)	cystolith（膀胱結石）	cyst(o)-「膀胱」
188	lith(o)-	G	ICF	体関連物質	石 (stone), 結石 (calculus)	lithogenous（結石生成性の）	-genous「〜を生じる」
189	-logist	G	FCF	医学・医療・学問	学者・専門家 (a person skilled in a branch of study)	ophthalmologist（眼科医）	ophthalm(o)-「目・眼」
190	-logy	G	FCF	医学・医療・学問	学問 (study of)	cardiology（心臓（病）学）	cardi(o)-「心臓」
191	lumb(o)-	L	ICF	体の部分	腰 (loin)	lumbosacral（腰仙の）	sacral「仙骨の・仙椎の」
192	lymph(o)-	L	ICF	心臓・血管・リンパ系	リンパ (lymph)	lymphocyte（リンパ球）	-cyte「細胞」
193	-lysis	G	FCF	医学・医療・学問	分解 (disintegration / decomposition)	analysis（分析）	ana-「上に」
194	macr(o)-	G	ICF	大小・形・色・数・量・状態・位置	大 (large)	macroadenoma（巨大腺腫）	adenoma「腺腫」
195	mal-	L	ICF	大小・形・色・数・量・状態・位置	悪・不良・異常 (bad / badly / wrong)	malpractice（医療過誤）	practice「（医師などの）実務・業務」
196	mamm(o)-	L	ICF	体の部分	乳房 (mamma / breast)	mammography（乳房撮影法）	-graphy「写法・記録法」
197	-mania	G	FCF	病気・症状	〜狂 (extreme obsession)	mythomania（虚言症）	mytho-「神話」
198	mast(o)-	G	ICF	体の部分	乳房 (breast), 乳頭 (nipple)	mastectomy（乳房切除）	-ectomy「切除（術）」
199	meg(a) / megal(o)-	G	ICF	大小・形・色・数・量・状態・位置	大 (large)	megacolon（巨大結腸症）	colon「結腸」
200	-megaly	L	FCF	病気・症状	肥大 (irregular enlargement)	cardiomegaly（心（臓）肥大（症））	cardi(o)-「心臓」
201	melan(o)-	G	ICF	大小・形・色・数・量・状態・位置	黒 (black), メラニン (melanin)	melanoma（黒色腫）	-oma「腫・瘤」

（次ページに続く）

(表1のつづき)

	接辞と連結形	語源	接辞と連結形の分類	関連分野	意味（英語）	用例（日本語）	用例解説
202	men(o)-	G	ICF	生殖器系	月経(menstruation)	dysmenorrhea / dysmenorrhoea（月経困難）	dys-「困難」, -rrhea / -rrhoea「排出・放出」
203	mening(o)-	G	ICF	脳神経系	髄膜(meninx)	meningocele（髄膜瘤・髄膜ヘルニア）	-cele「瘤・ヘルニア」
204	mes(o)-	G	ICF	大小・形・色・数・量・状態・位置	中(middle)	mesoappendix（虫垂間膜）	appendix「虫垂」
205	meta-	G	ICF	大小・形・色・数・量・状態・位置	変化(change)、～を超えた(beyond)、後ろ(behind)	metastasis（転移）	stasis「静止状態」
206	-meter	G	FCF	医学・医療・学問	計器・～計(instrument for measuring)	goniometer（角度計）	goni(o)-「角」
207	metr(o)-	G	ICF	生殖器系	子宮(uterus / womb)	metritis（子宮炎）(= uteritis / hysteritis)	-itis「～炎」
208	-metry	G	FCF	医学・医療・学問	測定(法)(measurement)	craniometry（頭蓋計測法）	crani(o)-「頭蓋(骨)」
209	micr(o)-	G	ICF	大小・形・色・数・量・状態・位置	小・微小(small)	microscope（顕微鏡）	-scope「見る器械」(⇔ macro-)
210	mid-	OE	ICF	大小・形・色・数・量・状態・位置	中間の(in the middle)	midbrain（中脳）	brain「脳」
211	mill(i)-	L	ICF	大小・形・色・数・量・状態・位置	1/1000 (one thousandth)	millimeter / millimetre（ミリメートル：1000分の1メートル）	ギリシャ語系の数は整数、ラテン語系の数は分数を表す
212	mis-	OE	ICF	大小・形・色・数・量・状態・位置	誤って・悪く(wrongly / badly)	miscarry（流産する）	carry「(子供を)身ごもっている」
213	mon(o)-	G	ICF	大小・形・色・数・量・状態・位置	1 (one / single)	monocyte（単球）	-cyte「細胞」
214	muc(o)- / muci-	L	ICF	体関連物質	粘液(mucus)	mucocutaneous（皮膚と粘膜の）	cutaneous「皮膚の」
215	mult(i)-	L	ICF	大小・形・色・数・量・状態・位置	多(much / many)	multifocal（多病巣性の）	focal「病巣の」
216	muscul(o)-	L	ICF	筋・骨格系	筋(肉)(muscle)	musculoskeletal（筋骨格の）	skeletal「骨格の」
217	my(o)-	G	ICF	筋・骨格系	筋(肉)(muscle)	myoatrophy（筋萎縮）	atrophy「萎縮」
218	myel(o)-	G	ICF	脳神経系	骨髄(bone marrow)、脊髄(spinal cord)	myeloma（骨髄腫）	-oma「腫・瘤」
219	nas(o)-	L	ICF	呼吸器系	鼻(nose)	nasopharyngitis（鼻咽頭炎）	pharyng(o)-「咽頭」, -itis「～炎」
220	necr(o)-	G	ICF	大小・形・色・数・量・状態・位置	死(death)	necropsy（検死）(=autopsy)	-opsy「検査」
221	neo-	G	ICF	大小・形・色・数・量・状態・位置	新しい(new)	neonatology（新生児学）	neonate「新生児」+ -o- + -logy「学問」
222	nephr(o)-	G	ICF	泌尿器系	腎臓(kidney)	nephropathy（腎臓病）	-pathy「病気」
223	neur(o)-	G	ICF	脳神経系	神経(nerve)、神経系(the nervous system)	neurocyte（神経細胞）	-cyte「細胞」
224	-nomy	G	FCF	医学・医療・学問	知識体系(system of knowledge regarding a field)	taxonomy（分類学）	tax(o)- / taxi-「順序・配列」
225	non-	L	Pref.	一般性が高い接頭辞	非(not)、消極的否定・欠如を示す	nonsmoking（禁煙の）	smoking「喫煙者用の・喫煙」
226	non(a)-	L	ICF	大小・形・色・数・量・状態・位置	9 (nine)	nonagon（九角形）	-gon「～角形」
227	null(i)-	L	ICF	大小・形・色・数・量・状態・位置	無(none / null)	nullify（無効にする）	-fy「～にする」
228	o(o)- / ov(o)- / ovi-	G	ICF	生殖器系	卵(egg)、卵子(ovum)	ovicide（殺卵剤）	-cide「～を殺す薬剤」
229	oct(a)- / oct(o)-	G/L	ICF	大小・形・色・数・量・状態・位置	8 (eight)	octagon（八角形）	-gon「～角形」
230	ocul(o)-	L	ICF	感覚器系	眼(eye)	oculometer（眼球運動測定器）	-meter「計器」

(次ページに続く)

(表1のつづき)

	接辞と連結形	語源	接辞と連結形の分類	関連分野	意味（英語）	用例（日本語）	用例解説
231	odont(o)-	G	ICF	消化器系	歯(tooth)	periodontitis(歯周炎)	peri-「周囲の」, -itis「〜炎」
232	-odynia	G	FCF	病気・症状	〜痛(pain)	pododynia(足底痛)	pod(o)-「足」
233	-oid	G	Suf.	一般性が高い接尾辞	〜に似た・〜のような(resembling / like)	arachnoid(クモ膜の)	arachn(o)-「クモ」
234	-ole	L	Suf.	一般性が高い接尾辞	小(small)	arteriole(小動脈、細動脈)	arteri(o)-「動脈」
235	olig(o)-	G	ICF	大小・形・色・数・量・状態・位置	少数・少量・欠乏(small / few / little)	oligospermia(精子減少症)	-spermia「〜な精子を有する状態」
236	om(o)-	G	ICF	体の部分	肩(shoulder)	omohyoid(肩甲舌骨の)	hyoid「舌骨の」
237	-oma	G	Suf.	病気・症状	腫・瘤(tumor)	adenoma(腺腫)	aden(o)-「腺」
238	omni-	L	ICF	一般性が高い接頭辞	全(all)	omnipresent(遍在する)	omni- + praesens「存在する（ラテン語）」より
239	onco-	G	ICF	病気・症状	腫瘍(tumor)	oncology(腫瘍学)	-logy「学問」
240	oophor(o)-	L	ICF	生殖器系	卵巣(ovary)	oophorectomy(卵巣切除(術))	-ectomy「切除(術)」
241	ophthalm(o)-	G	ICF	感覚器系	眼(eye)	ophthalmology(眼科学)	-logy「学問」
242	-opia	G	FCF	医学・医療・学問	視力障害(visual disorder)	diplopia(複視・二重視)	dipl(o)-「複〜・二重〜」
243	-opsia / -opsy	G	FCF	医学・医療・学問	見ること(viewing)	myodesopsia(飛蚊症)、biopsy(生検)	muioeides「蚊のように（ギリシャ語）」+ -opsia, bi(o)-「生・生命・生物」
244	-or	L	Suf.	一般性が高い接尾辞	〜する人（もの）(a person or thing that performs the action described by the verb)	governor(統治者)	govern「統治する」
245	or(o)-	L	ICF	消化器系	口(mouth)	oral(口頭の・経口の・口で行う)	-al 接尾辞「〜の」
246	orchi(o) / orchid(o)-	G	ICF	生殖器系	睾丸・精巣(testis / testicle)	orchitis(睾丸炎)	-itis「〜炎」
247	-orexia	G	FCF	医学・医療・学問	欲望(desire)、食欲(appetite)	anorexia(食欲不振・無食欲)、anorexia nervosa(神経性食欲不振，拒食症)	a- / an-「不・無・非」
248	orth(o)-	G	ICF	大小・形・色・数・量・状態・位置	まっすぐな(straight)、正しい(right)	orthopedics / orthopaedics(整形外科)	orthos「まっすぐな・正しい（ギリシャ語）」+ paideia「子供の養育・教育（ギリシャ語）」
249	-osis	G	Suf.	病気・症状	病的状態(abnormal condition)	narcosis(昏睡状態)	narc(o)-「麻痺・麻酔・睡眠」
250	oste(o)-	G	ICF	筋・骨格系	骨(bone)	osteoma(骨腫)	-oma「腫・瘤」
251	ot(o)-	G	ICF	感覚器系	耳(ear)	otoscope(耳鏡)	-scope「見る器械」
252	ot(o)-	G	ICF	体の部分	耳(ear)	otolith(耳石)	-lith「石」
253	ov(o)-	L	ICF	生殖器系	卵(egg)、卵子(ovum)	ovogenesis(卵形成)	-genesis「発生」
254	ovari(o)-	L	ICF	生殖器系	卵巣(ovary)	ovariectomy(卵巣切除(術))	-ectomy「切除(術)」
255	over-	OE	Pref.	一般性が高い接頭辞	過度の(excessively)、上方に(upper)	overactive bladder(過活動膀胱)	bladder「膀胱(urinary bladder)」
256	palat(o)-	L	ICF	消化器系	口蓋(palate)	palatal(口蓋の)	-al 接尾辞「〜の」
257	pale(o)-	G	ICF	大小・形・色・数・量・状態・位置	古・旧(ancient)	paleobiology(古生物学)	biology「生物学」
258	pan-	G	ICF	大小・形・色・数・量・状態・位置	全(all)、総(universal)	pandemic(全国(世界)的流行の)	pan- + demos「人々（ギリシャ語）」+ -ic「〜の：接尾辞」cf. epidemic

（次ページに続く）

(表1のつづき)

	接辞と連結形	語源	接辞と連結形の分類	関連分野	意味(英語)	用例(日本語)	用例解説
259	pancreat(o)-	G	ICF	消化器系	膵臓(pancreas)	pancreatotomy(膵臓切開(術))	-tomy「切開(術)」
260	para-¹	G	Pref.	一般性が高い接頭辞	側に(beside)	paramedical(医療補助的な)	medical「医療の」
261	para-²	G	Pref.	病気・症状	異常(abnormal), 欠陥(defective)	parakinesia(運動錯誤)	-kinesia「運動」
262	path(o)-	G	ICF	病気・症状	病気(disease)	pathology(病理学)	-logy「学問」
263	-pathy	G	FCF	病気・症状	感情(feeling), 苦痛(suffering), 病気・〜症(disorder / disease), 療法(treatment)	neuropathy(神経障害), apathy(無感動・無関心)	neur(o)-「神経」, a-「不・無・非」
264	ped(o)- / pod(o)- / pedi-	L	ICF	体の部分	足(foot)	podiatry(足病学・足病治療)(= chiropody)	-iatry「医療」
265	pelv(o)- / pelvi-	L	ICF	筋・骨格系	骨盤(pelvis)	pelvic(骨盤の)	-ic「〜の・〜に関する」
266	-penia	G	FCF	病気・症状	欠乏(deficiency)	sarcopenia(筋肉減少症)	sarc(o)-「肉」
267	pent(a)-	G	ICF	大小・形・色・数・量・状態・位置	5(five)	pentadactyl(5本の指を持った)	-dactyl(= -dactylous)「〜の指を有する」
268	-pepsia	G	FCF	医学・医療・学問	消化(digestion)	dyspepsia(消化不良)	dys-「困難な」
269	per-	L	Pref.	一般性が高い接頭辞	〜を通して(through / all over)	permanent(永久の)	per- + *manere*「残る(ラテン語)」
270	peri-	G	Pref.	一般性が高い接頭辞	まわりの(around / about)	perineuritis(神経周膜炎)	neur(o)-「神経」, -itis「〜炎」
271	-pexy	G	FCF	医学・医療・学問	固定(surgical fixation)	enteropexy(腸固定術)	enter(o)-「腸」
272	-phagia / -phagy	G	FCF	病気・症状	食べること(eating)	dysphagia(嚥下障害)	dys-「困難な」
273	phall(o)-	G	ICF	生殖器系	陰茎(penis)	phalloplasty(陰茎形成(手術))	-plasty「形成(手術)」
274	pharmac(o)-	G	ICF	医学・医療・学問	薬(drug)	pharmacotherapy(薬物療法)	therapy「療法」
275	pharyng(o)-	G	ICF	呼吸器系	咽頭(pharynx)	pharyngitis(咽頭炎)	-itis「〜炎」
276	-phasia	G	FCF	病気・症状	言語障害(speech disorder)	dysphasia(不全失語症)	dys-「困難な」
277	-philia	G	FCF	病気・症状	〜の病的愛好(unnatural attraction)	pedophilia(小児性愛)	ped(o)- / paed(o)-「子供」
278	phleb(o)-	G	ICF	心臓・血管・リンパ系	静脈(vein)	phlebolysis(静脈内注入)(= venoclysis)	clysis「注液・注入」
279	-phobia	G	FCF	病気・症状	恐怖症(extreme fear)	acrophobia(高所恐怖症)	acr(o)-「先端」
280	phon(o)-	G	ICF	自然界の諸要素	音(sound)	phonocardiograph(心音計)	cardiograph「心拍記録器」
281	phot(o)-	G	ICF	自然界の諸要素	光(light), 写真(photograph)	photodermatitis(光線皮膚炎)	dermatitis「皮膚炎」
282	phren(o)-	G	ICF	呼吸器系	横隔膜(diaphragm)	phrenic(横隔膜の)	-ic「〜の・〜に関する」
283	-phrenia	G	FCF	病気・症状	精神障害(mental disorder)	schizophrenia(統合失調症)	schiz(o)-「分裂」
284	physi(o)-	G	ICF	医学・医療・学問	物理学の(physical), 生理学の(physiological), 天然の(natural)	physiotherapy(理学療法)(= physical therapy)	therapy「治療・療法」
285	-phyte	G	FCF	病気・症状	増殖体(growth)	osteophyte(骨棘・骨増殖体)	oste(o)-「骨」
286	-plasm	G	FCF	医学・医療・学問	形成するもの(formative substance)	cytoplasm(細胞質)	cyt(o)-「細胞」

(次ページに続く)

(表1のつづき)

	接辞と連結形	語源	接辞と連結形の分類	関連分野	意味（英語）	用例（日本語）	用例解説
287	-plasty	G	FCF	医学・医療・学問	形成（手術）(surgical repair)	mammoplasty / mammaplasty（乳房形成術）	mamm(o)- / mamma「乳房」
288	-plegia	G	FCF	病気・症状	麻痺 (paralysis)	hemiplegia（半側麻痺）	hemi-「半」
289	pleur(o)-	G	ICF	呼吸器系	肋膜・胸膜 (pleura)	pleural（肋膜の・胸膜の）	-al 接尾辞「〜の」
290	-pnea / -pnoea	G	FCF	医学・医療・学問	呼吸 (breathing)	hyperpnea / hyperpnoea（過呼吸）	hyper-「過度の」 cf. dyspnea, apnea, eupnea
291	pneumon(o)- / pneum(o)-	G	ICF	呼吸器系	肺 (lung)	pneumococcus（肺炎球菌）	coccus「球菌」
292	-poiesis	G	FCF	医学・医療・学問	産出 (production), 形成 (formation)	hematopoiesis / hemopoiesis（造血・血液生成）	hemat(o)- / hem(o)-「血」
293	poly-	G	ICF	大小・形・色・数・量・状態・位置	多 (much / many)	polyarthritis（多発関節炎）	arthritis「関節炎」
294	poro-	G	ICF	大小・形・色・数・量・状態・位置	細穴・孔 (pore)	osteoporosis（骨粗鬆症）	oste(o)-「骨」, -osis「病的状態」
295	post-	L	Pref.	一般性が高い接頭辞	後の (after / behind)	postoperative（手術後の）	operative「手術の」（⇔ ante- / pre-）
296	-praxia	G	FCF	医学・医療・学問	動作 (action)	apraxia（失行（症）・行動障害）	a- / an-「不・無・非」
297	pre-	L	Pref.	一般性が高い接頭辞	〜前の・〜の前にある (before)	preoperative（手術前の）	operative「手術の」（⇔ post-）
298	pro-	G	Pref.	一般性が高い接頭辞	前・前〜 (before)	prognosis（予後）	-gnosis「認識」 cf. diagnosis
299	proct(o)-	G	ICF	消化器系	肛門 (anus), 直腸 (rectum)	proctologist（肛門科医）	-logist「〜の研究者」
300	pros-	G	Pref.	大小・形・色・数・量・状態・位置	〜に加えて (in addition)	prosthesis（人工装具）	*prostithenai*（ギリシャ語, pros + tithenai「置く」）
301	prostat(o)-	G	ICF	生殖器系	前立腺 (prostate)	prostatotomy（前立腺切開（術））	-tomy「切開（術）」
302	pseud(o)-	G	ICF	大小・形・色・数・量・状態・位置	偽 (false)	pseudoarthrosis（偽関節）(=false joint)	arthrosis「関節症」
303	psych(o)-	G	ICF	人間一般	精神 (mind)	psychiatry（精神医学）	-iatry「医療」
304	pulmon(o)- / pulmoni-	L	ICF	呼吸器系	肺 (lung)	pulmonary（肺の，肺疾患の）	-ary 接尾辞「〜に関する・〜の」
305	py(o)-	G	ICF	体関連物質	うみ・膿汁 (pus)	pyoderma（膿皮症）	-derma「皮膚病」
306	pyel(o)-	G	ICF	泌尿器系	腎盂 (renal pelvis)	pyelitis（腎盂炎）	-itis「〜炎」
307	pylor(o)-	G	ICF	消化器系	幽門 (pylorus)	pyloroplasty（幽門形成）	-plasty「形成（手術）」
308	pyr(o)-	G	ICF	自然界の諸要素	火 (fire)	pyrogen（発熱物質）	-gen「〜を生じるもの」
309	quadr(i)- / quart-	L	ICF	大小・形・色・数・量・状態・位置	4 (four)	quadriplegia（四肢麻痺）	-plegia「麻痺」
310	quinqu(e)- / quint(i)-	L	ICF	大小・形・色・数・量・状態・位置	5 (five)	quinquecentennial（500年間）	centennial「100周年」
311	radi(o)-	L	ICF	筋・骨格系	橈骨 (radius)	radiocarpal（橈骨手根骨の）	carpal「手根（骨）の」
312	radi(o)-	L	ICF	自然界の諸要素	放射線 (radiation)	radiodermatitis（放射線皮膚炎）	dermatitis「皮膚炎」
313	re-	L	Pref.	一般性が高い接頭辞	再 (again / anew)	recuperate（回復する）	*recuperare*（ラテン語, re- + capere「取る」）
314	rect(o)-	L	ICF	消化器系	直腸 (rectum)	rectoscope（直腸鏡）	-scope「見る器械」
315	reni- / reno-	L	ICF	泌尿器系	腎臓 (kidney)	reniform（腎臓形の）	-form「〜の形を持つ」
316	retin(o)-	L	ICF	感覚器系	網膜 (retina)	retinopathy（網膜症）	-pathy「病気」

(次ページに続く)

(表1のつづき)

	接辞と連結形	語源	接辞と連結形の分類	関連分野	意味（英語）	用例（日本語）	用例解説
317	retro-	L	Pref.	一般性が高い接頭辞	後方の・後方へ (behind / backward)	retrocecal（盲腸後方の）	cecal「盲腸（cecum）の」
318	rhin(o)-	G	ICF	呼吸器系	鼻 (nose)	rhinitis（鼻炎）	-itis「〜炎」
319	rhin(o)-	G	ICF	体の部分	鼻 (nose)	rhinopharyngitis（鼻咽頭炎）	pharyng(o)-「咽頭」、-itis「〜炎」
320	-rrhage	G	FCF	病気・症状	異常流出 (excessive and abnormal flow)	hemorrhage（大出血）	hem(o)-「血」
321	-rrhagia	G	FCF	病気・症状	異常流出 (excessive and abnormal flow)	meningorrhagia（髄膜出血）	mening(o)-「髄膜」
322	-rrhaphy	G	FCF	医学・医療・学問	縫合 (suture)	enterorrhaphy（腸縫合術）	enter(o)-「腸」
323	-rrhea / -rrhoea	G	FCF	病気・症状	流出 (discharge / flow)	diarrhea（下痢）	dia-「〜を通じて・〜を横切って」
324	-rrhexis	G	FCF	病気・症状	破裂 (rupture)	arteriorrhexis（動脈破裂）	arteri(o)-「動脈」
325	sacr(o)-	L	ICF	筋・骨格系	仙骨 (sacrum)	sacroiliac（仙骨と腸骨の）	iliac「腸骨の」
326	salping(o)-	G	ICF	生殖器系	卵管 (salpinx / Fallopian tube)	salpingitis（卵管炎）	-itis「〜炎」
327	sarc(o)-	G	ICF	体関連物質	肉 (flesh)	sarcoma（肉腫）	-oma「腫・瘤」
328	scapul(o)-	L	ICF	筋・骨格系	肩甲骨 (scapula)	scapuloclavicular（肩甲骨と鎖骨の）	clavicular「鎖骨（clavicle）の」
329	-schisis	G	FCF	病気・症状	亀裂 (fissure)	palatoschisis（口蓋裂）	palato-「口蓋」
330	schiz(o)-	G	ICF	大小・形・色・数・量・状態・位置	分裂 (split)	schizophrenia（統合失調症）	-phrenia「精神障害」
331	scler(o)-	G	ICF	大小・形・色・数・量・状態・位置	固い (hard)	sclerosis（硬化（症））	-osis「病的状態」
332	-scope	G	FCF	医学・医療・学問	見る器械 (instrument to view)	endoscope（内視鏡）	end(o)-「内（部）」
333	-scopic	G	FCF	医学・医療・学問	観察の (pertaining to visual examination)	endoscopic（内視鏡検査の）	end(o)-「内（部）」
334	-scopy	G	FCF	医学・医療・学問	検査・観察 (process of visual examination)	endoscopy（内視鏡検査（法））	end(o)-「内（部）」
335	semi-	L	Pref.	一般性が高い接頭辞	半〜 (half)、部分的に (partly)	semicoma（半昏睡）	coma「昏睡」cf. hemi-（ギリシャ語）
336	sept(i)-	L	ICF	大小・形・色・数・量・状態・位置	7 (seven)	septangle（七角形）	angle「角」
337	ser(o)-	L	ICF	心臓・血管・リンパ系	血清 (serum)	serodiagnosis（血清学的診断）	diagnosis「診断」
338	sex(i)-	L	ICF	大小・形・色・数・量・状態・位置	6 (six)	sexangular（六角形の）	(= hexagonal)
339	sial(o)-	G	ICF	体関連物質	唾液 (saliva)	sialorrhea（流涎症・唾液分泌過多）	-rrhea「流出」
340	somat(o)-	G	ICF	体の部分	身体 (body)	somatometry（生体計測）	-metry「測定（法）」
341	son(o)- / soni-	L	ICF	自然界の諸要素	音 (sound)	sonograph（ソノグラフ・音波検査機）(= ultrasonograph)	-graph「記録計器」
342	sperm(o)- / spermi- / spermat(o)-	G	ICF	体関連物質	精子・精液 (sperm / semen)	spermatorrhea（精液漏）	-rrhea「流出」
343	sphygm(o)-	G	ICF	心臓・血管・リンパ系	脈拍 (pulse)	sphygmomanometer（血圧計）	manometer「圧力計・血圧計」
344	spin(o)- / spini-	L	ICF	筋・骨格系	脊柱 (spinal column)、脊髄 (spinal cord)、とげ (spine)	spinal（背骨の・脊柱の・脊髄の）	-al 接尾辞「〜の」
345	spir(o)-	L	ICF	呼吸器系	呼吸 (breathing)	spirometry（肺活量測定（法））	-metry「測定法」
346	splen(o)-	G	ICF	心臓・血管・リンパ系	脾臓 (spleen)	splenectomy（脾臓切除術）	-ectomy「切除（術）」

（次ページに続く）

(表1のつづき)

	接辞と連結形	語源	接辞と連結形の分類	関連分野	意味（英語）	用例（日本語）	用例解説
347	-stasis	G	FCF	医学・医療・学問	停止 (stopping)	homeostasis(恒常性)	home(o)-「類似の」
348	sten(o)-	G	ICF	大小・形・色・数・量・状態・位置	狭い (narrow)	stenosis(狭窄)	-osis「病的状態」
349	stern(o)-	G	ICF	筋・骨格系	胸骨 (sternum)	sternoclavicular(胸骨と鎖骨の)	clavicular「鎖骨 (clavicle) の」
350	stomat(o)-	G	ICF	消化器系	口 (mouth)	stomatology(口腔病学)	-logy「学問」
351	-stomy	G	FCF	医学・医療・学問	開口術 (forming a new opening)	gastrostomy(胃造瘻術)	gastr(o)-「胃」
352	sub-	L	Pref.	一般性が高い接頭辞	下に (below), 下の (under)	subarachnoid(くも膜下の)	arachn(o)-「蜘蛛・くも膜」, -oid「～状の(もの)」
353	super-	L	Pref.	一般性が高い接頭辞	上位・過度の (above / over / beyond)	superabduction(過外転)	abduction「外転」
354	supra-	L	Pref.	一般性が高い接頭辞	上の・上に (above / beyond)	suprascapular(肩甲骨上の)	scapular「肩甲骨の」
355	sur-	L	Pref.	一般性が高い接頭辞	上に・上を (over / above)	surpass(～にまさる・凌ぐ)	*surpasser*(中世フランス語)より, sur- + *passer*「超える」
356	syn- / sym-	G	Pref.	一般性が高い接頭辞	共に・同時に・似た (with / together)	syndrome(症候群)	-drome「走る, 競走路」
357	tacho-	G	ICF	大小・形・色・数・量・状態・位置	速度 (speed)	tachometer(回転速度計・流速計)	-meter「～計」
358	tachy-	G	ICF	大小・形・色・数・量・状態・位置	速い (rapid / swift)	tachycardia(頻脈)	-cardia「心臓活動」
359	tele-	G	ICF	大小・形・色・数・量・状態・位置	遠距離の (at a distance)	telesurgery(遠隔手術)	surgery「手術」
360	teno-	G	ICF	筋・骨格系	腱 (tendon)	tenodesis(腱固定(術))	-desis「束縛」
361	tetr(a)-	G	ICF	大小・形・色・数・量・状態・位置	4 (four)	tetraplegia(四肢麻痺)	-plegia「麻痺」(= quadriplegia)
362	therm(o)-	G	ICF	自然界の諸要素	熱 (heat)	thermometer(温度計・体温計)	-meter「計器」
363	thorac(o)-	G	ICF	体の部分	胸 (thorax / chest)	thoracocentesis(胸腔穿刺)	centesis「穿刺」
364	thromb(o)-	G	ICF	心臓・血管・リンパ系	血液凝固の (relating to blood clotting)	thrombocyte(血小板) (= blood platelet)	-cyte「細胞」
365	thyr(o)-	G	ICF	内分泌系	甲状腺 (thyroid)	thyroidectomy(甲状腺切除(術))	-ectomy「切除(術)」
366	tibio-	L	ICF	筋・骨格系	脛骨 (tibia) と～の	tibiofibular(脛腓骨の)	fibular「腓骨の」
367	-tome	G	FCF	医学・医療・学問	切断具 (instrument for cutting), 切片 (segment)	microtome(ミクロトーム)	micro-「小・微小」
368	tomo-	G	ICF	大小・形・色・数・量・状態・位置	切断 (cut), 部分 (section)	tomography(断層撮影法)	-graphy「写法」
369	-tomy	G	FCF	医学・医療・学問	切開(術) (cutting)	gastrotomy(胃切開(術))	gastr(o)-「胃」
370	-tonia	L	FCF	病気・症状	緊張の状態 (condition of tention)	myotonia(筋緊張(症))	my(o)-「筋(肉)」
371	tonsill(o)-	L	ICF	心臓・血管・リンパ系	扁桃 (tonsil)	tonsillar(扁桃腺の)	-ar 接尾辞「～の」
372	tox(o)- / toxi- / toxic(o)-	G	ICF	自然界の諸要素	毒 (poison / toxic)	toxemia of pregnancy(妊娠中毒症)	-emia / -aemia「～な血液を有する状態」
373	trache(o)-	L	ICF	呼吸器系	気管 (trachea)	tracheobronchial(気管と気管支の)	bronchial「気管支の」
374	trans-	L	Pref.	一般性が高い接頭辞	横切って・越えて・貫いて (across / beyond / through)	transcortical(皮質間の)	cortical「皮質の・皮質性の」
375	tri-	G/L	ICF	大小・形・色・数・量・状態・位置	3 (three), 3倍の・3重の (threefold)	triplegia(三肢麻痺)	-plegia「麻痺」
376	trich(o)-	G	ICF	体関連物質	毛・毛髪 (hair)	trichogenous(発毛の)	-genous「～を生じる」

(次ページに続く)

（表1のつづき）

	接辞と連結形	語源	接辞と連結形の分類	関連分野	意味（英語）	用例（日本語）	用例解説
377	tripl(o)-	G	ICF	大小・形・色・数・量・状態・位置	3倍の・3重の (threefold)	triploblastic（三胚葉性の）	-blastic「～な胚の」
378	-trophy	G	FCF	医学・医療・学問	栄養(nourishment), 成長(growth)	dystrophy（栄養障害/発育異常/筋萎縮）	dys-「困難な」
379	ulno-	L	ICF	筋・骨格系	尺骨(ulna)	ulnocarpal（尺骨手根の）	carpal「手根の」
380	ultra-	L	Pref.	一般性が高い接頭辞	超・～を超えた (beyond)	ultramicrotome（超ミクロトーム）	microtome「顕微鏡用剥片切断機」, micro-「微・小」, -tome「切断器具」
381	un-	OE	Pref.	一般性が高い接頭辞	否定(not)	unable（～することができない）	able「～することができる」
382	under-	OE	Pref.	一般性が高い接頭辞	下に(below), 不十分に(insufficiently)	underestimate（過小評価する）	estimate「評価する」
383	uni-	L	ICF	大小・形・色・数・量・状態・位置	1(one / single)	unicellular（単細胞の）	cellular「細胞の」
384	ur(o)-	G	ICF	体関連物質	尿(urine), 排尿(urination)	urology（泌尿器学）	-logy「学問」
385	ureter(o)-	G	ICF	泌尿器系	尿管(ureter)	ureterolithotomy（尿管切開術）	lithotomy「切石術・砕石術」
386	urethr(o)-	G	ICF	泌尿器系	尿道(urethra)	urethral（尿道の）	-al 接尾辞「～の」
387	-uria	G	FCF	病気・症状	尿の状態 (urinary condition)	hematuria（血尿(症)）	hemat(o)-「血」
388	uter(o)-	L	ICF	生殖器系	子宮(uterus / womb)	uteralgia（子宮痛）(= metralgia・hysteralgia)	-algia「～痛」
389	vagin(o)-	L	ICF	生殖器系	腟(vagina)	vaginitis（腟炎）(= colpitis)	-itis「～炎」
390	vas(o)-	L	ICF	心臓・血管・リンパ系	脈管(vessel), 血管(blood vessel)	vasodilator（血管拡張薬）	dilator「拡張薬」
391	vascul(o)-	L	ICF	心臓・血管・リンパ系	血管(blood vessel)	cardiovascular（心臓血管の）	cardi(o)-「心臓」
392	ven(o)-	L	ICF	心臓・血管・リンパ系	静脈(vein)	venography（静脈造影法）(= phlebography)	-graphy「写法」
393	viscer(o)- / visceri-	L	ICF	体の部分	内臓の(visceral)	viscerotropic（内臓向性の）	-tropic「向～性の」
394	xanth(o)-	G	ICF	大小・形・色・数・量・状態・位置	黄(yellow)	xanthoma（黄色腫）	-oma「腫・瘤」

表2　医学用語―語頭要素(接頭辞・前部連結形)分野別一覧

	接辞と連結形	語源	接辞と連結形の分類	分野	意味(英語)	用例(日本語)	用例解説
1	acromi(o)-	L	ICF	筋・骨格系	肩峰(acromion)	acromioclavicular(肩峰鎖骨の)	clavicular「鎖骨の」
2	arthr(o)-	G	ICF	筋・骨格系	関節(joint)	arthritis(関節炎)	-itis「〜炎」
3	carp(o)-	G	ICF	筋・骨格系	手根(wrist)	radiocarpal(橈骨手根骨の)	radi(o)-「橈骨」
4	chondr(o)- / chondri-	G	ICF	筋・骨格系	軟骨(cartilage)	chondrocyte(軟骨細胞)	-cyte「細胞」
5	clavi- / clav(o)-	L	ICF	筋・骨格系	鎖骨(clavicle)	clavipectoral fascia(鎖骨胸筋筋膜)	pectoral「胸筋の」, fascia「筋膜」
6	cost(o)-	L	ICF	筋・骨格系	肋骨(rib)	costectomy(肋骨切除)	-ectomy「切除(術)」
7	crani(o)-	G	ICF	筋・骨格系	頭蓋骨(cranium)	craniometry(頭蓋骨計測法)	-metry「測定法」
8	humer(o)-	L	ICF	筋・骨格系	上腕(骨)(humerus)の	humeral(上腕骨の)	-al 接尾辞「〜の」
9	ili(o)-	L	ICF	筋・骨格系	腸骨(ilium)	iliofemoral(腸骨と大腿骨の)	femoral「大腿骨の」
10	ischi(o)-	G	ICF	筋・骨格系	坐骨(ischium)	ischial(坐骨の)	-al 接尾辞「〜の」
11	muscul(o)-	L	ICF	筋・骨格系	筋(肉)(muscle)	musculoskeletal(筋骨格の)	skeletal「骨格の」
12	my(o)-	G	ICF	筋・骨格系	筋(肉)(muscle)	myoatrophy(筋萎縮)	atrophy「萎縮」
13	oste(o)-	G	ICF	筋・骨格系	骨(bone)	osteoma(骨腫)	-oma「腫・瘤」
14	pelv(o)- / pelvi-	L	ICF	筋・骨格系	骨盤(pelvis)	pelvic(骨盤の)	-ic「〜の・〜に関する」
15	radi(o)-	L	ICF	筋・骨格系	橈骨(radius)	radiocarpal(橈骨手根骨の)	carpal「手根(骨)の」
16	sacr(o)-	L	ICF	筋・骨格系	仙骨(sacrum)	sacroiliac(仙骨と腸骨の)	iliac「腸骨の」
17	scapul(o)-	L	ICF	筋・骨格系	肩甲骨(scapula)	scapuloclavicular(肩甲骨と鎖骨の)	clavicular「鎖骨(clavicle)の」
18	spin(o)- / spini-	L	ICF	筋・骨格系	脊柱(spinal column), 脊髄(spinal cord), とげ(spine)	spinal(背骨の・脊柱・脊髄の)	-al 接尾辞「〜の」
19	stern(o)-	G	ICF	筋・骨格系	胸骨(sternum)	sternoclavicular(胸骨と鎖骨の)	clavicular「鎖骨(clavicle)の」
20	teno-		ICF	筋・骨格系	腱(tendon)	tenodesis(腱固定(術))	-desis「束縛」
21	tibio-	L	ICF	筋・骨格系	脛骨(tibia)と〜の	tibiofibular(脛腓骨の)	fibular「腓骨の」
22	ulno-	L	ICF	筋・骨格系	尺骨(ulna)	ulnocarpal(尺骨手根の)	carpal「手根の」
23	angi(o)-	G	ICF	心臓・血管・リンパ系	血管(blood vessel)	angioma(血管腫)	-oma「腫, 瘤」
24	aort(o)-	G	ICF	心臓・血管・リンパ系	大動脈(aorta)	aortitis(大動脈炎)	-it is「〜炎」
25	arteri(o)-	G	ICF	心臓・血管・リンパ系	動脈(artery)	arteriosclerosis(動脈硬化症)	sclerosis「硬化症」
26	blast(o)-	L	ICF	心臓・血管・リンパ系	胚(embryo), 芽(sprout / germ)	blastoma(芽腫)	-oma「腫・瘤」
27	cardi(o)-	G	ICF	心臓・血管・リンパ系	心臓(heart), 噴門(cardia)	cardiologist(心臓病専門医)	-logist「〜の研究者」
28	hemat(o)- / haemat(o)- / hem(o)- / haem(o)- / hema- / haema-	G	ICF	心臓・血管・リンパ系	血液(blood)	hematology(血液学)	-logy「学問」

(次ページに続く)

(表2のつづき)

	接辞と連結形	語源	接辞と連結形の分類	分野	意味(英語)	用例(日本語)	用例解説
29	leuc(o)- / leuk(o)-	G	ICF	心臓・血管・リンパ系	白(white), 白血球(leucocyte / leukocyte)	leukemia / leukaemia (白血病)	-emia / -aemia「血液の状態」cf. erythrocyte, thrombocyte
30	lymph(o)-	L	ICF	心臓・血管・リンパ系	リンパ(lymph)	lymphocyte(リンパ球)	-cyte「細胞」
31	phleb(o)-	G	ICF	心臓・血管・リンパ系	静脈(vein)	phleboclysis(静脈内注入)(= venoclysis)	clysis「注液・注入」
32	ser(o)-	L	ICF	心臓・血管・リンパ系	血清(serum)	serodiagnosis(血清学的診断)	diagnosis「診断」
33	sphygm(o)-	G	ICF	心臓・血管・リンパ系	脈拍(pulse)	sphygmomanometer(血圧計)	manometer「圧力計・血圧計」
34	splen(o)-	G	ICF	心臓・血管・リンパ系	脾臓(spleen)	splenectomy(脾臓切除術)	-ectomy「切除(術)」
35	thromb(o)-	G	ICF	心臓・血管・リンパ系	血液凝固の(relating to blood clotting)	thrombocyte(血小板)(= blood platelet)	-cyte「細胞」
36	tonsill(o)-	L	ICF	心臓・血管・リンパ系	扁桃(tonsil)	tonsillar(扁桃腺の)	-ar 接尾辞「~の」
37	vas(o)-	L	ICF	心臓・血管・リンパ系	脈管(vessel), 血管(blood vessel)	vasodilator(血管拡張薬)	dilator「拡張薬」
38	vascul(o)-	L	ICF	心臓・血管・リンパ系	血管(blood vessel)	cardiovascular(心臓血管の)	cardi(o)-「心臓」
39	ven(o)-	L	ICF	心臓・血管・リンパ系	静脈(vein)	venography(静脈造影法)(= phlebography)	-graphy「写法」
40	append(o)- / appendic(o)-	L	ICF	消化器系	虫垂(appendix)	appendectomy / appendicectomy(虫垂切除術)	-ectomy「切除(術)」
41	cheil(o)- / chil(o)-	G	ICF	消化器系	唇(lip)	cheilotomy(口唇切開術)	-tomy「切開(術)」
42	cholecyst(o)-	L	ICF	消化器系	胆嚢(gallbladder / cholecyst)	cholecystitis(胆嚢炎)	-itis「~炎」
43	col(o)-	G	ICF	消化器系	結腸(colon)	colectomy(結腸切除)	-ectomy「切除(術)」
44	dent(o)- / denti-	L	ICF	消化器系	歯(tooth)	dental(歯の)	-al 接尾辞「~の」
45	duoden(o)-	L	ICF	消化器系	十二指腸(duodenum)	duodenal ulcer(十二指腸潰瘍)	-al 接尾辞「~の」
46	enter(o)-	G	ICF	消化器系	腸(intestine)	enterobacteria(腸内細菌)	bacteria「細菌(bacterium)」の複数形
47	esophag(o)- / oesophag(o)-	G	ICF	消化器系	食道(esophagus / oesophagus)	esophagitis / oesophagitis(食道炎)	-itis「~炎」
48	gastr(o)-	G	ICF	消化器系	胃(stomach)	gastralgia(胃痛)	-algia「~痛」
49	gingiv(o)-	L	ICF	消化器系	歯肉(gum)	gingivitis(歯肉炎)	-itis「~炎」
50	gloss(o)-	L	ICF	消化器系	舌(tongue)	glossoplegia(舌麻痺)	-plegia「麻痺」
51	hepat(o)-	G	ICF	消化器系	肝臓(liver)	hepatitis(肝炎)	-itis「~炎」
52	ile(o)-	L	ICF	消化器系	回腸(ileum)	ileocolitis(回結腸炎)	-col(o)「結腸」, -itis「~炎」
53	jejun(o)-	L	ICF	消化器系	空腸(jejunum)	jejunostomy(空腸造瘻術)	-stomy「開口術」
54	labi(o)-	L	ICF	消化器系	唇(lip)	labiodental(唇歯音の)	dental「歯音の」
55	odont(o)-	G	ICF	消化器系	歯(tooth)	periodontitis(歯周炎)	peri-「周囲の」, -itis「~炎」
56	or(o)-	L	ICF	消化器系	口(mouth)	oral(口頭の・経口の・口で行う)	-al 接尾辞「~の」
57	palat(o)-	L	ICF	消化器系	口蓋(palate)	palatal(口蓋の)	-al 接尾辞「~の」
58	pancreat(o)-	G	ICF	消化器系	膵臓(pancreas)	pancreatotomy(膵臓切開(術))	-tomy「切開(術)」

(次ページに続く)

(表2のつづき)

	接辞と連結形	語源	接辞と連結形の分類	分野	意味(英語)	用例(日本語)	用例解説
59	proct(o)-	G	ICF	消化器系	肛門(anus), 直腸(rectum)	proctologist(肛門科医)	-logist「〜の研究者」
60	pylor(o)-	G	ICF	消化器系	幽門(pylorus)	pyloroplasty(幽門形成)	-plasty「形成(手術)」
61	rect(o)-	L	ICF	消化器系	直腸(rectum)	rectoscope(直腸鏡)	-scope「見る器械」
62	stomat(o)-	G	ICF	消化器系	口(mouth)	stomatology(口腔病学)	-logy「学問」
63	alveol(o)-	L	ICF	呼吸器系	肺胞・歯槽(alveolus)	alveolitis(肺胞炎)	-itis「〜炎」
64	bronch(o)- / bronchi(o)-	G	ICF	呼吸器系	気管支(bronchus)	bronchoscope(気管支鏡)	-scope「見る器械」
65	laryng(o)-	G	ICF	呼吸器系	喉頭(larynx)	laryngotomy(喉頭切開)	-tomy「切開(術)」
66	nas(o)-	L	ICF	呼吸器系	鼻(nose)	nasopharyngitis(鼻咽頭炎)	pharyng(o)-「咽頭」, -itis「〜炎」
67	pharyng(o)-	G	ICF	呼吸器系	咽頭(pharynx)	pharyngitis(咽頭炎)	-itis「〜炎」
68	phren(o)-	G	ICF	呼吸器系	横隔膜(diaphragm)	phrenic(横隔膜の)	-ic「〜の・〜に関する」
69	pleur(o)-	G	ICF	呼吸器系	肋膜・胸膜(pleura)	pleural(肋膜の・胸膜の)	-al 接尾辞「〜の」
70	pneumon(o)- / pneum(o)-	G	ICF	呼吸器系	肺(lung)	pneumococcus(肺炎球菌)	coccus「球菌」
71	pulmon(o)- / pulmoni-	L	ICF	呼吸器系	肺(lung)	pulmonary(肺の, 肺疾患の)	-ary 接尾辞「〜に関する・〜の」
72	rhin(o)-	G	ICF	呼吸器系	鼻(nose)	rhinitis(鼻炎)	-itis「〜炎」
73	spir(o)-	L	ICF	呼吸器系	呼吸(breathing)	spirometry(肺活量測定(法))	-metry「測定法」
74	trache(o)-	L	ICF	呼吸器系	気管(trachea)	tracheobronchial(気管と気管支の)	bronchial「気管支の」
75	cyst(o)-	G	ICF	泌尿器系	膀胱(urinary bladder)	cystolith(膀胱結石)	-lith「結石」
76	nephr(o)-	G	ICF	泌尿器系	腎臓(kidney)	nephropathy(腎臓病)	-pathy「病気」
77	pyel(o)-	G	ICF	泌尿器系	腎盂(renal pelvis)	pyelitis(腎盂炎)	-itis「〜炎」
78	reni- / reno-	L	ICF	泌尿器系	腎臓(kidney)	reniform(腎臓形の)	-form「〜の形を持つ」
79	ureter(o)-	G	ICF	泌尿器系	尿管(ureter)	ureterolithotomy(尿管切石術)	lithotomy「切石術・砕石術」
80	urethr(o)-	G	ICF	泌尿器系	尿道(urethra)	urethral(尿道の)	-al 接尾辞「〜の」
81	colp(o)-	G	ICF	生殖器系	腟(vagina)	colpitis(腟炎)(= vaginitis)	-itis「〜炎」
82	episio-	G	ICF	生殖器系	外陰(vulva)	episiotomy(会陰切開(術))	-tomy「〜切開(術)」
83	hyster(o)-	G	ICF	生殖器系	子宮(uterus / womb)	hysterotomy(子宮切開)	-tomy「切開(術)」
84	men(o)-	G	ICF	生殖器系	月経(menstruation)	dysmenorrhea / dysmenorrhoea(月経困難)	dys-「困難」, -rrhea / -rrhoea「排出・放出」
85	metr(o)-	G	ICF	生殖器系	子宮(uterus / womb)	metritis(子宮炎)(= uteritis / hysteritis)	-itis「〜炎」
86	o(o)- / ov(o)- / ovi-	G	ICF	生殖器系	卵(egg), 卵子(ovum)	ovicide(殺卵剤)	-cide「〜を殺す薬剤」
87	oophor(o)-	L	ICF	生殖器系	卵巣(ovary)	oophorectomy(卵巣切除(術))	-ectomy「切除(術)」
88	orchi(o)- / orchid(o)-	G	ICF	生殖器系	睾丸・精巣(testis / testicle)	orchitis(睾丸炎)	-itis「〜炎」

(次ページに続く)

(表2のつづき)

	接辞と連結形	語源	接辞と連結形の分類	分野	意味(英語)	用例(日本語)	用例解説
89	ov(o)-	L	ICF	生殖器系	卵(egg), 卵子(ovum)	ovogenesis(卵形成)	-genesis「発生」
90	ovari(o)-	L	ICF	生殖器系	卵巣(ovary)	ovariectomy(卵巣切除(術))	-ectomy「切除(術)」
91	phall(o)-	G	ICF	生殖器系	陰茎(penis)	phalloplasty(陰茎形成(手術))	-plasty「形成(手術)」
92	prostat(o)-	G	ICF	生殖器系	前立腺(prostate)	prostatotomy(前立腺切開(術))	-tomy「切開(術)」
93	salping(o)-	G	ICF	生殖器系	卵管(salpinx / Fallopian tube)	salpingitis(卵管炎)	-itis「〜炎」
94	uter(o)-	L	ICF	生殖器系	子宮(uterus / womb)	uteralgia(子宮痛)(=metralgia / hysteralgia)	-algia「〜痛」
95	vagin(o)-	L	ICF	生殖器系	腟(vagina)	vaginitis(腟炎)(= colpitis)	-itis「〜炎」
96	thyr(o)-	G	ICF	内分泌系	甲状腺(thyroid)	thyroidectomy(甲状腺切除(術))	-ectomy「切除(術)」
97	cerebell(o)- / cerebelli-	L	ICF	脳神経系	小脳(cerebellum)	cerebellar(小脳の)	-ar 接尾辞「〜の」
98	cerebr(o)-	L	ICF	脳神経系	脳(brain), 大脳(cerebrum)	cerebrospinal(脳脊髄の)	spinal「背骨の・脊髄の」
99	encephal(o)-	G	ICF	脳神経系	脳(brain)	encephalocele(脳ヘルニア)	-cele「ヘルニア」
100	gangli(o)-	G	ICF	脳神経系	神経節(ganglion)	ganglioma(神経節腫)	-oma「腫・瘤」
101	mening(o)-	G	ICF	脳神経系	髄膜(meninx)	meningocele(髄膜瘤・髄膜ヘルニア)	-cele「瘤・ヘルニア」
102	myel(o)-	G	ICF	脳神経系	骨髄(bone marrow), 脊髄(spinal cord)	myeloma(骨髄腫)	-oma「腫・瘤」
103	neur(o)-	G	ICF	脳神経系	神経(nerve), 神経系(the nervous system)	neurocyte(神経細胞)	-cyte「細胞」
104	alg(o)-	G	ICF	感覚器系	〜痛(pain)	algometry(痛覚検査)	-metry「測定(法)」
105	audi(o)-	L	ICF	感覚器系	聴覚(hearing), 音(sound)	audiometry(聴力測定)	-metry「測定(法)」
106	aur(i)-	L	ICF	感覚器系	耳(ear)	aural(耳の)	-al 接尾辞「〜の」
107	cerat(o)- / kerat(o)-	G	ICF	感覚器系	角膜(cornea)	keratitis(角膜炎)	-itis「〜炎」
108	dermat(o)- / derma- / derm(o)-	G	ICF	感覚器官	皮膚(skin)	dermatology(皮膚科学)	-logy「学問」
109	kerat(o)- / cerat(o)-	G	ICF	感覚器系	角膜(cornea)	keratitis(角膜炎)	-itis「〜炎」
110	ocul(o)-	L	ICF	感覚器系	眼(eye)	oculometer(眼球運動測定器)	-meter「計器」
111	ophthalm(o)-	G	ICF	感覚器系	眼(eye)	ophthalmology(眼科学)	-logy「学問」
112	ot(o)-	G	ICF	感覚器系	耳(ear)	otoscope(耳鏡)	-scope「見る器械」
113	retin(o)-	L	ICF	感覚器系	網膜(retina)	retinopathy(網膜症)	-pathy「病気」
114	abdomin(o)-	L	ICF	体の部分	腹部(abdomen)	abdominal(腹部の)	-al 接尾辞「〜の」
115	brachi(o)-	L	ICF	体の部分	腕(arm), 上腕(upper arm)	brachialgia(上腕痛)	-algia「〜痛」
116	cephal(o)-	G	ICF	体の部分	頭部(head)	cephalomegaly(頭部巨大症)	-megaly「(〜の部分の)巨大(症)」
117	cervic(o)-	L	ICF	体の部分	首・頸部(neck / cervix)	cervicography(子宮頸管撮影)	-graphy「写法」
118	cortic(o)-	L	ICF	体の部分	(大脳/副腎)皮質(cortex)	corticosteroid(コルチコステロイド)	steroid「ステロイド」

(次ページに続く)

(表2のつづき)

	接辞と連結形	語源	接辞と連結形の分類	分野	意味(英語)	用例(日本語)	用例解説
119	dactyl(o)-	G	ICF	体の部分	指(finger)	dactyloscopy(指紋検査)	-scopy「検査・観察」
120	dors(o)- / dorsi-	L	ICF	体の部分	背(back)	dorsolateral(背部側部の)	lateral「側面の」
121	lapar(o)-	G	ICF	体の部分	脇腹(flank),腹壁(abdominal wall)	laparoscope(腹腔鏡)	-scope「見る器械」
122	laryng(o)-	G	ICF	体の部分	喉頭(larynx)	laryngotomy(喉頭切開)	-tomy「切開(術)」
123	lumb(o)-	L	ICF	体の部分	腰(loin)	lumbosacral(腰仙の)	sacral「仙骨の, 仙椎の」
124	mamm(o)-	L	ICF	体の部分	乳房(mamma / breast)	mammography(乳房撮影法)	-graphy「写法, 記録法」
125	mast(o)-	G	ICF	体の部分	乳房(breast),乳頭(nipple)	mastectomy(乳房切除)	-ectomy「切除(術)」
126	om(o)-	G	ICF	体の部分	肩(shoulder)	omohyoid(肩甲舌骨の)	hyoid「舌骨の」
127	ot(o)-	G	ICF	体の部分	耳(ear)	otolith(耳石)	-lith「石」
128	ped(o)- / pod(o)- / pedi-	L	ICF	体の部分	足(foot)	podiatry(足病学・足病治療)(= chiropody)	-iatry「医療」
129	rhin(o)-	G	ICF	体の部分	鼻(nose)	rhinopharyngitis(鼻咽頭炎)	pharyng(o)-「咽頭」, -itis「〜炎」
130	somat(o)-	G	ICF	体の部分	身体(body)	somatometry(生体計測)	-metry「測定(法)」
131	thorac(o)-	G	ICF	体の部分	胸(thorax / chest)	thoracocentesis(胸腔穿刺)	centesis「穿刺」
132	viscer(o)- / visceri-	L	ICF	体の部分	内臓の(visceral)	viscerotropic(内臓向性の)	-tropic「向〜性の」
133	aden(o)-	G	ICF	体関連物質	腺(gland)	adenocarcinoma(腺癌)	carcinoma「癌腫」
134	albumin(o)-	L	ICF	体関連物質	蛋白(albumin)	albuminous(アルブミン・蛋白の)	-ous「〜を持つ・〜の特徴を有する」
135	chol(o)- / chole-	G	ICF	体関連物質	胆汁(bile / gall)	cholelith(胆石)	-lith「結石」
136	cyt(o)-	G	ICF	体関連物質	細胞(cell)	cytoplasm(細胞質)	-plasm「形成するもの」
137	fibr(o)-	L	ICF	体関連物質	線維(fiber)	fibroadenoma(線維腺腫)	adenoma「腺腫」
138	glyc(o)- / gluc(o)-	G	ICF	体関連物質	糖(sugar)	glycogen(グリコーゲン)	-gen「〜を生じるもの」
139	hidr(o)-	G	ICF	体関連物質	汗(sweat)	hidrosis(過剰発汗)	-osis「病的状態」
140	lact(o)-	L	ICF	体関連物質	乳(milk)	lactoprotein(乳蛋白質)	protein「蛋白」
141	lip(o)-	G	ICF	体関連物質	脂肪(fat)	lipocyte(脂肪細胞)	-cyte「細胞」
142	lith(o)-	G	ICF	体関連物質	石(stone),結石(calculus)	lithogenous(結石生成性の)	-genous「〜を生じる」
143	muc(o)- / muci-	L	ICF	体関連物質	粘液(mucus)	mucocutaneous(皮膚と粘膜の)	cutaneous「皮膚の」
144	py(o)-	G	ICF	体関連物質	うみ・膿汁(pus)	pyoderma(膿皮症)	-derma「皮膚病」
145	sarc(o)-	G	ICF	体関連物質	肉(flesh)	sarcoma(肉腫)	-oma「腫・瘤」
146	sial(o)-	G	ICF	体関連物質	唾液(saliva)	sialorrhea(流涎症・唾液分泌過多)	-rrhea「流出」
147	sperm(o)- / spermi- / spermat(o)-	G	ICF	体関連物質	精子・精液(sperm / semen)	spermatorrhea(精液漏)	-rrhea「流出」
148	trich(o)-	G	ICF	体関連物質	毛・毛髪(hair)	trichogenous(発毛の)	-genous「〜を生じる」

(次ページに続く)

（表2のつづき）

	接辞と連結形	語源	接辞と連結形の分類	分野	意味（英語）	用例（日本語）	用例解説
149	ur(o)-	G	ICF	体関連物質	尿(urine), 排尿(urination)	urology(泌尿器学)	-logy「学問」
150	carcin(o)-	G	ICF	病気・症状	癌(cancer)	carcinogen(発癌物質)	-gen「〜を生むもの」
151	onco-	G	ICF	病気・症状	腫瘍(tumor)	oncology(腫瘍学)	-logy「学問」
152	para-²	G	Pref.	病気・症状	異常(abnormal), 欠陥(defective)	parakinesia(運動錯誤)	-kinesia「運動」
153	path(o)-	G	ICF	病気・症状	病気(disease)	pathology(病理学)	-logy「学問」
154	chem(o)-	L	ICF	医学・医療・学問	化学の(chemical)	chemotherapy(化学療法)	therapy「治療」
155	electr(o)-			医学・医療・学問	電気(electricity)	electrocardiography(心電図検査)	cardiography「心拍記録(法)」
156	pharmac(o)-	G	ICF	医学・医療・学問	薬(drug)	pharmacotherapy(薬物療法)	therapy「療法」
157	physi(o)-			医学・医療・学問	物理学の(physical), 生理学の(physiological), 天然の(natural)	physiotherapy(理学療法)(= physical therapy)	therapy「治療・療法」
158	acr(o)-	G	ICF	大小・形・色・数・量・状態・位置	先端・頂上(top / peak / summit)	acrophobia(高所恐怖症)	-phobia「恐怖症」
159	anis(o)-	G	ICF	大小・形・色・数・量・状態・位置	不等(unequal)	anisodactylous(不等指症の)	dactyl-「指／足指」
160	aut(o)-	G	ICF	大小・形・色・数・量・状態・位置	自己(self), 自動の(by itself)	autoantibody(自己抗体)	antibody「抗体」
161	bi-	L	ICF	大小・形・色・数・量・状態・位置	2(two / double)	bisexual(両性素質の)	sexual「性の」
162	brady-	G	ICF	大小・形・色・数・量・状態・位置	遅い(slow)	bradykinesia(動作緩慢)	-kinesia「運動」
163	cent(i)-	L	ICF	大小・形・色・数・量・状態・位置	1/100(one hundredth)	centimeter / centimetre(センチメートル)	ギリシャ語系の数は整数、ラテン語系の数は分数を表す
164	chlor(o)-	G	ICF	大小・形・色・数・量・状態・位置	緑(green)	chlorophyl(葉緑素)	-phyl(l)「植物内の〜色素」
165	chrom(o)- / chromat(o)-	G	ICF	大小・形・色・数・量・状態・位置	色(color)	chromatopsia(色視症：物が異常に着色されてみえる状態)	-opsia「〜視」
166	cyan(o)-	G	ICF	大小・形・色・数・量・状態・位置	藍(dark blue)	cyanosis(チアノーゼ)	-osis「病的状態」
167	dec(a)-	G	ICF	大小・形・色・数・量・状態・位置	10(ten)	decagon(十角形)	-gon「〜角形」
168	deci-	L	ICF	大小・形・色・数・量・状態・位置	10分の1(one tenth)	deciliter / decilitre(デシリットル)	liter / litre「リットル(容量の単位)」
169	dextr(o)-	L	ICF	大小・形・色・数・量・状態・位置	右(right)	dextrocardia(右胸心)	-cardia「心臓の働き・位置」
170	dipl(o)-	G	ICF	大小・形・色・数・量・状態・位置	2(two / double)	diplococcus(双球菌)	coccus「球菌」
171	dist(o)-	L	ICF	大小・形・色・数・量・状態・位置	末端の・遠位の(distal)	distal(遠位の)	-al 接尾辞「〜の」
172	dys-	G	ICF	大小・形・色・数・量・状態・位置	悪化(bad), 困難な(difficult)	dyspnea(呼吸困難)	-pnea / -pnoea「呼吸」
173	ect(o)-	G	ICF	大小・形・色・数・量・状態・位置	外の(external)	ectocornea(角膜上皮)	cornea「角膜」
174	end(o)-	G	ICF	大小・形・色・数・量・状態・位置	内部(within)	endoscopy(内視鏡検査)	-scopy「検査・観察」
175	ennea-		ICF	大小・形・色・数・量・状態・位置	9(nine)	enneagon(九角形)	-gon「〜角形」
176	equi-	L	ICF	大小・形・色・数・量・状態・位置	等しい(equal)	equicaloric(等カロリーの)	caloric「カロリーの」
177	erythr(o)-	G	ICF	大小・形・色・数・量・状態・位置	赤(red), 赤血球(erythrocyte)	erythrocyte(赤血球)	-cyte「細胞」cf. leukocyte(白血球), thrombocyte(血小板)

（次ページに続く）

（表2のつづき）

	接辞と連結形	語源	接辞と連結形の分類	分野	意味（英語）	用例（日本語）	用例解説
178	eu-	G	ICF	大小・形・色・数・量・状態・位置	良（well / good）	eupnea（正常呼吸）	-pnea / -pnoea「呼吸」
179	fore-	OE	ICF	大小・形・色・数・量・状態・位置	前の（the front part of / before）	forearm（前腕），forehead（額）	arm「腕」，head「頭」
180	geront(o)-	G	ICF	大小・形・色・数・量・状態・位置	老人（old man），老齢（old age）	gerontology（老人学・老年学）	-logy「学問」
181	glauc(o)-	G	ICF	大小・形・色・数・量・状態・位置	緑灰色の（bluish-grey）	glaucoma（緑内障）	*glaukoma*「水晶体の濁り（ギリシャ語）」より
182	hect(o)-	G	ICF	大小・形・色・数・量・状態・位置	100（hundred）	hectare（ヘクタール：100アールに相当）	ギリシャ語系の数は整数，ラテン語系の数は分数を表す
183	hemi-	G	ICF	大小・形・色・数・量・状態・位置	半分（half）	hemiplegia（半側麻痺）	-plegia「麻痺」
184	hept(a)-	G	ICF	大小・形・色・数・量・状態・位置	7（seven）	heptahedron（七面体）	-hedron「〜面体」
185	heter(o)-	G	ICF	大小・形・色・数・量・状態・位置	異（different）	heterogenous（外来の・外生の）	-genous「〜によって発生する／〜を生じる」
186	hex(a)-	G	ICF	大小・形・色・数・量・状態・位置	6（six）	hexahedron（六面体）	-hedron「〜面体」
187	hom(o)-	G	ICF	大小・形・色・数・量・状態・位置	同（same）	homosexual（同性愛の）	sexual「性の」
188	is(o)-	G	ICF	大小・形・色・数・量・状態・位置	等（equal）	isogenic（同質遺伝子型の）	-genic「遺伝子の」
189	kil(o)-	G	ICF	大小・形・色・数・量・状態・位置	1000（thousand）	kilogram（キログラム）	ギリシャ語系の数は整数，ラテン語系の数は分数を表す
190	kinesi(o)-	G	ICF	大小・形・色・数・量・状態・位置	動き（movement）	kinesitherapy / kinesiotherapy（運動療法）	therapy「治療・療法」
191	leuc(o)- / leuk(o)-	G	ICF	大小・形・色・数・量・状態・位置	白（white），白血球（leucocyte / leukocyte）	leukemia / leukaemia（白血病）	-emia / -aemia「血液の状態」 cf. erythrocyte, thrombocyte
192	macr(o)-	G	ICF	大小・形・色・数・量・状態・位置	大（large）	macroadenoma（巨大腺腫）	adenoma「腺腫」
193	mal-	L	ICF	大小・形・色・数・量・状態・位置	悪・不良・異常（bad / badly / wrong）	malpractice（医療過誤）	practice「（医師などの）実務・業務」
194	meg(a)/ megal(o)-	G	ICF	大小・形・色・数・量・状態・位置	大（large）	megacolon（巨大結腸症）	colon「結腸」
195	melan-	G	ICF	大小・形・色・数・量・状態・位置	黒（black），メラニン（melanin）	melanoma（黒色腫）	-oma「腫・瘤」
196	mes(o)-	G	ICF	大小・形・色・数・量・状態・位置	中（middle）	mesoappendix（虫垂間膜）	appendix「虫垂」
197	meta-	G	ICF	大小・形・色・数・量・状態・位置	変化（change）〜を超えた（beyond），後ろ（behind）	metastasis（転移）	stasis「静止状態」
198	micr(o)-	G	ICF	大小・形・色・数・量・状態・位置	小・微小（small）	microscope（顕微鏡）	-scope「見る器械」（⇔ macro-）
199	mid-	OE	ICF	大小・形・色・数・量・状態・位置	中間の（in the middle）	midbrain（中脳）	brain「脳」
200	mill(i)-	L	ICF	大小・形・色・数・量・状態・位置	1/1000（one thousandth）	millimeter / millimetre（ミリメートル：1000分の1メートル）	ギリシャ語系の数は整数，ラテン語系の数は分数を表す
201	mis-	OE	ICF	大小・形・色・数・量・状態・位置	誤って・悪く（wrongly / badly）	miscarry（流産する）	carry「（子供を）身ごもっている」
202	mon(o)-	G	ICF	大小・形・色・数・量・状態・位置	1（one / single）	monocyte（単球）	-cyte「細胞」
203	mult(i)-	L	ICF	大小・形・色・数・量・状態・位置	多（much / many）	multifocal（多病巣性の）	focal「病巣の」
204	necr(o)-	G	ICF	大小・形・色・数・量・状態・位置	死（death）	necropsy（検死）（= autopsy）	-opsy「検査」
205	neo-	G	ICF	大小・形・色・数・量・状態・位置	新しい（new）	neonatology（新生児学）	neonate「新生児」+ -o- + -logy「学問」
206	non(a)-	L	ICF	大小・形・色・数・量・状態・位置	9（nine）	nonagon（九角形）	-gon「〜角形」

（次ページに続く）

（表2のつづき）

	接辞と連結形	語源	接辞と連結形の分類	分野	意味(英語)	用例(日本語)	用例解説
207	null(i)-	L	ICF	大小・形・色・数・量・状態・位置	無(none / null)	nullify(無効にする)	-fy「～にする」
208	oct(a)- / oct(o)-	G/L	ICF	大小・形・色・数・量・状態・位置	8(eight)	octagon(八角形)	-gon「～角形」
209	olig(o)-	G	ICF	大小・形・色・数・量・状態・位置	少数・少量・欠乏(small / few / little)	oligospermia(精子減少症)	-spermia「～な精子を有する状態」
210	orth(o)-	G	ICF	大小・形・色・数・量・状態・位置	まっすぐな(straight), 正しい(right)	orthopedics / orthopaedics(整形外科)	*orthos*「まっすぐな・正しい(ギリシャ語)」+ *paideia*「子供の養育・教育(ギリシャ語)」
211	pale(o)-	G	ICF	大小・形・色・数・量・状態・位置	古・旧(ancient)	paleobiology(古生物学)	biology「生物学」
212	pan-	G	ICF	大小・形・色・数・量・状態・位置	全(all), 総(universal)	pandemic(全国(世界)的流行の)	pan- + *demos*「人々(ギリシャ語)」+ -ic「～の：接尾辞」cf. epidemic
213	pent(a)-	G	ICF	大小・形・色・数・量・状態・位置	5(five)	pentadactyl(5本の指を持った)	-dactyl(= -dactylous)「～の指を有する」
214	poly-	G	ICF	大小・形・色・数・量・状態・位置	多(much / many)	polyarthritis(多発関節炎)	arthritis「関節炎」
215	poro-	G	ICF	大小・形・色・数・量・状態・位置	細穴・孔(pore)	osteoporosis(骨粗鬆症)	oste(o)-「骨」, -osis「病的状態」
216	pros-	G	Pref.	大小・形・色・数・量・状態・位置	～に加えて(in addition)	prosthesis(人工装具)	*prostithenai*「ギリシャ語, pros + *tithenai*「置く」
217	pseud(o)-	G	ICF	大小・形・色・数・量・状態・位置	偽(false)	pseudoarthrosis(偽関節 = false joint)	arthrosis「関節症」
218	quadr(i)- / quart-	L	ICF	大小・形・色・数・量・状態・位置	4(four)	quadriplegia(四肢麻痺)	-plegia「麻痺」
219	quinqu(e)- / quint(i)-	L	ICF	大小・形・色・数・量・状態・位置	5(five)	quinquecentennial(500年間)	centennial「100周年」
220	schiz(o)-	G	ICF	大小・形・色・数・量・状態・位置	分裂(split)	schizophrenia(統合失調症)	-phrenia「精神障害」
221	scler(o)-	G	ICF	大小・形・色・数・量・状態・位置	固い(hard)	sclerosis(硬化(症))	-osis「病的状態」
222	sept(i)-	L	ICF	大小・形・色・数・量・状態・位置	7(seven)	septangle(七角形)	angle「角」
223	sex(i)-	L	ICF	大小・形・色・数・量・状態・位置	6(six)	sexangular(六角形の)	(= hexagonal)
224	sten(o)-	G	ICF	大小・形・色・数・量・状態・位置	狭い(narrow)	stenosis(狭窄)	-osis「病的状態」
225	tacho-	G	ICF	大小・形・色・数・量・状態・位置	速度(speed)	tachometer(回転速度計・流速計)	-meter「～計」
226	tachy-	G	ICF	大小・形・色・数・量・状態・位置	速い(rapid / swift)	tachycardia(頻脈)	-cardia「心臓活動」
227	tele-	G	ICF	大小・形・色・数・量・状態・位置	遠距離の(at a distance)	telesurgery(遠隔手術)	surgery「手術」
228	tetr(a)-	G	ICF	大小・形・色・数・量・状態・位置	4(four)	tetraplegia(四肢麻痺)	-plegia「麻痺」(= quadriplegia)
229	tomo-	G	ICF	大小・形・色・数・量・状態・位置	切断(cut), 部分(section)	tomography(断層撮影法)	-graphy「写法」
230	tri-	G/L	ICF	大小・形・色・数・量・状態・位置	3(three), 3倍の・3重の(threefold)	triplegia(三肢麻痺)	-plegia「麻痺」
231	tripl(o)-	G	ICF	大小・形・色・数・量・状態・位置	3倍の・3重の(threefold)	triploblastic(三胚葉性の)	-blastic「～な胚の」
232	uni-	L	ICF	大小・形・色・数・量・状態・位置	1(one / single)	unicellular(単細胞の)	cellular「細胞の」
233	xanth(o)-	G	ICF	大小・形・色・数・量・状態・位置	黄(yellow)	xanthoma(黄色腫)	-oma「腫・瘤」
234	dem(o)-	G	ICF	人間一般	人々(people)	demography(人口統計学)	-graphy「記述法」
235	immun(o)-	L	ICF	人間一般	免疫(immunity)	immunodeficiency(免疫不全)	deficiency「欠乏・不足」
236	lingu(o)- / lingui-	L	ICF	人間一般	言語(language), 舌(tongue)	linguistic(言語の)	-istic 形容詞をつくる接尾辞「～の」

（次ページに続く）

(表2のつづき)

	接辞と連結形	語源	接辞と連結形の分類	分野	意味（英語）	用例（日本語）	用例解説
237	psych(o)-	G	ICF	人間一般	精神(mind)	psychiatry（精神医学）	-iatry「医療」
238	aer(o)-	G	ICF	自然界の諸要素	空気(air)	aerophagia（空気嚥下）	-phagia / -phagy「食べること」
239	aqua- / aqui-	L	ICF	自然界の諸要素	水(water)	aqueous（水の・水溶性の・水を含む）	-eous 接尾辞「～の性質を持つ」
240	bi(o)-	G	ICF	自然界の諸要素	生命(life)	biopsy（生検）	-opsy「見ること」⇒「検査」
241	eco-	G	ICF	自然界の諸要素	生態(学)(ecology)	ecosystem（生態系）	system「系」
242	gynec(o)- / gynaec(o)-	G	ICF	自然界の諸要素	女性(woman)	gynecology / gynaecology（婦人科学）	-logy「学問」
243	hydr(o)-	G	ICF	自然界の諸要素	水(water)	hydrocephalus（水頭症）	-cephalus「頭部異常」
244	phon(o)-	G	ICF	自然界の諸要素	音(sound)	phonocardiograph（心音計）	cardiograph「心拍記録器」
245	phot(o)-	G	ICF	自然界の諸要素	光(light)，写真(photograph)	photodermatitis（光線皮膚炎）	dermatitis「皮膚炎」
246	pyr(o)-	G	ICF	自然界の諸要素	火(fire)	pyrogen（発熱物質）	-gen「～を生じるもの」
247	radi(o)-	L	ICF	自然界の諸要素	放射線(radiation)	radiodermatitis（放射線皮膚炎）	dermatitis「皮膚炎」
248	son(o)- / soni-	L	ICF	自然界の諸要素	音(sound)	sonograph（ソノグラフ・音波検査機）（= ultrasonograph）	-graph「記録計器」
249	therm(o)-	G	ICF	自然界の諸要素	熱(heat)	thermometer（温度計・体温計）	-meter「計器」
250	tox(o)- / toxi- / toxic(o)-	G	ICF	自然界の諸要素	毒(poison / toxic)	toxemia of pregnancy（妊娠中毒症）	-emia / -aemia「～な血液を有する状態」
251	a- / an-	G	Pref.	一般性が高い接頭辞	不・無・非(not / without)	apnea（無呼吸）	-pnea / -pnoea「呼吸」
252	ab-	L	Pref.	一般性が高い接頭辞	～から離れた(away from)	abnormal（異常な）	normal「標準の・正常の」
253	ana-	G	Pref.	一般性が高い接頭辞	上・後・再(up / back / again)	analysis（分析）	-lysis「分解」
254	ante-	L	Pref.	一般性が高い接頭辞	前の(before)	antebrachial（前腕の）	brachial「腕の」(⇔ post-)
255	anti-	G	Pref.	一般性が高い接頭辞	反・対・抗(against / preventing)	antibacterial（抗菌性の）	bacterial「細菌の」
256	circum-	L	Pref.	一般性が高い接頭辞	周囲に・取り巻く(around)	circumoral（口腔周囲の）	oral「口(腔)の」
257	co-	L	Pref.	一般性が高い接頭辞	共同の・相互の・副(jointly / mutually)	cocarcinogen（発癌補助物質）	carcinogen「発癌物質」
258	contra-	L	Pref.	一般性が高い接頭辞	反対・逆(against / opposite)	contraception（避妊）	contra- +(con)ception「妊娠，受胎」
259	crypt(o)-	G	ICF	一般性が高い接頭辞	隠された(hidden)	cryptogenic（原因不明の）	-genic「～を生み出す・遺伝子を有する」
260	de-	L	Pref.	一般性が高い接頭辞	分離(away)，下降(down from)	deform（～の形を損なう）	form「形づくる」
261	di-	G	Pref.	一般性が高い接頭辞	2 (two / twice / double)	dioxide（二酸化物）	oxide「酸化物」
262	dia-	G	Pref.	一般性が高い接頭辞	通して・横切って・離れて(through / across / apart)	diagnosis（診断）	-gnosis「認識」
263	dis-	L	Pref.	一般性が高い接頭辞	不・無・非(not / opposite of / absence of)	disability（障害・無能）	ability「能力」
264	em-	L	Pref.	一般性が高い接頭辞	中に入れる(put into)，～の状態にする(bring into the condition of)	embalm（死体に防腐処置をする）	balm「芳香性樹脂」

(次ページに続く)

(表2のつづき)

	接辞と連結形	語源	接辞と連結形の分類	分野	意味（英語）	用例（日本語）	用例解説
265	en-	L	Pref.	一般性が高い接頭辞	中に入れる（put into），～の状態にする（bring into the condition of）	enrich（富ませる）	rich「金持ちの・豊かな」
266	epi-	G	Pref.	一般性が高い接頭辞	上（upon / above）	epidemic（流行性の・流行(病)）	epi- + *demos*「人々（ギリシャ語）」+ -ic「～の：接尾辞」cf. pandemic
267	ex-	G	Pref.	一般性が高い接頭辞	外に（out）	excrete（排出する・分泌する）	*excerenere*「排出する（ラテン語）」より，ex-「外へ」+ *cerenere*「篩にかける・より分ける」
268	exo-	G	Pref.	一般性が高い接頭辞	外（external / from outside）	exocrine（外分泌（性）の）	exo- + *crine*「分離する（ギリシャ語）」(⇔ endocrine)
269	extra-	L	Pref.	一般性が高い接頭辞	～外の（outside / beyond）	extracarpal（手根外の）	carpal「手根(骨)の」
270	hyp(o)-	G	Pref.	一般性が高い接頭辞	下の・不足の（below / deficient）	hypoacidity（低酸症）	acidity「酸(性)度」(⇔ hyper-)
271	hyper-	G	Pref.	一般性が高い接頭辞	過度の（over / excessive）	hyperpnea（過呼吸）	-pnea / -pnoea「呼吸」
272	il-	L	Pref.	一般性が高い接頭辞	不・無・非（not）	illegal（違法の）	legal（適法の）
273	im-	L	Pref.	一般性が高い接頭辞	不・無・非（not）	impossible（不可能な）	possible「可能な」
274	in-¹	L	Pref.	一般性が高い接頭辞	中へ（into）	include（含む）	*includere*「囲む・閉じ込める（ラテン語）」より，in- + *claudere*「閉じる」
275	in-²	L	Pref.	一般性が高い接頭辞	不・無・非（not）	infertility（生殖不能）	fertility「受胎能力」
276	infra-	L	Pref.	一般性が高い接頭辞	下に・～の下の（below）	infraclavicular（鎖骨下の）	clavicular「鎖骨（clavicle）の」
277	inter-	L	Pref.	一般性が高い接頭辞	間・相互の（between / among）	intervertebral（脊椎間の）	vertebral「脊椎の」
278	intra-	L	Pref.	一般性が高い接頭辞	内の（within / inside）	intravascular（血管内の）	vascular「血管の」
279	intro-	L	Pref.	一般性が高い接頭辞	中に（to the inside）	introvert（内向性の）	intro- + *vertere*「回転する・向く」
280	ir-	L	Pref.	一般性が高い接頭辞	不・無・非（not）	irregular（不規則な）	regular（規則的な）
281	non-	L	Pref.	一般性が高い接頭辞	非（not），消極的否定・欠如を示す	nonsmoking（禁煙の）	smoking「喫煙者用の・喫煙」
282	omni-	L	ICF	一般性が高い接頭辞	全（all）	omnipresent（遍在する）	omni- + *praesens*「存在する（ラテン語）」より
283	over-	OE	Pref.	一般性が高い接頭辞	過度の（excessively），上方に（upper）	overactive bladder（過活動膀胱）	bladder「膀胱（urinary bladder）」
284	para-¹	G	Pref.	一般性が高い接頭辞	側に（beside）	paramedical（医療補助的な）	medical「医療の」
285	per-	L	Pref.	一般性が高い接頭辞	～を通して（through / all over）	permanent（永久の）	per- + *manere*「残る（ラテン語）」
286	peri-	G	Pref.	一般性が高い接頭辞	まわりの（around / about）	perineuritis（神経周膜炎）	neur(o)-「神経」，-itis「～炎」
287	post-	L	Pref.	一般性が高い接頭辞	後の（after / behind）	postoperative（手術後の）	operative「手術の」(⇔ ante- / pre-)
288	pre-	L	Pref.	一般性が高い接頭辞	～前の・～の前にある（before）	preoperative（手術前の）	operative「手術の」(⇔ post-)
289	pro-	G	Pref.	一般性が高い接頭辞	前・前へ（before）	prognosis（予後）	-gnosis「認識」cf. diagnosis
290	re-	L	Pref.	一般性が高い接頭辞	再（again / anew）	recuperate（回復する）	*recuperare*（ラテン語，re- + *capere*「取る」）
291	retro-	L	Pref.	一般性が高い接頭辞	後方の・後方へ（behind / backward）	retrocecal（盲腸後方の）	cecal「盲腸（cecum）の」
292	semi-	L	Pref.	一般性が高い接頭辞	半～（half），部分的に（partly）	semicoma（半昏睡）	coma「昏睡」cf. *hemi*-（ギリシャ語）
293	sub-	L	Pref.	一般性が高い接頭辞	下に（below），下の（under）	subarachnoid（くも膜下の）	arachn(o)-「蜘蛛・くも膜」，-oid「～状の(もの)」

（次ページに続く）

(表2のつづき)

	接辞と連結形	語源	接辞と連結形の分類	分野	意味(英語)	用例(日本語)	用例解説
294	super-	L	Pref.	一般性が高い接頭辞	上位・過度の(above / over / beyond)	superabduction(過外転)	abduction「外転」
295	supra-	L	Pref.	一般性が高い接頭辞	上の・上に(above / beyond)	suprascapular(肩甲骨上の)	scapular「肩甲骨の」
296	sur-	L	Pref.	一般性が高い接頭辞	上に・上を(over / above)	surpass(〜にまさる・凌ぐ)	*surpasser*(中世フランス語, sur- + *passer*(pass)
297	syn- / sym-	G	Pref.	一般性が高い接頭辞	共に・同時に・似た(with / together)	syndrome(症候群)	-drome「走る・競走路」
298	trans-	L	Pref.	一般性が高い接頭辞	横切って・越えて・貫いて(across / beyond / through)	transcortical(皮質間の)	cortical「皮質の・皮質性の」
299	ultra-	L	Pref.	一般性が高い接頭辞	超・〜を超えた(beyond)	ultramicrotome(超ミクロトーム)	microtome「顕微鏡用剝片切断機」, micro-「微・小」, -tome「切断器具」
300	un-	OE	Pref.	一般性が高い接頭辞	否定(not)	unable(〜することができない)	able「〜することができる」
301	under-	OE	Pref.	一般性が高い接頭辞	下に(below), 不十分に(insufficiently)	underestimate(過小評価する)	estimate「評価する」

表3　医学用語―語末要素(接尾辞・後部連結形)分野別一覧

	接辞と連結形	語源	接辞と連結形の分類	分野	意味(英語)	用例(日本語)	用例解説
1	-iasis	G	Suf.	病気・症状	〜性の病気(forming names of disorders)	psoriasis(乾癬)	*psora*「かゆみ(ギリシャ語)」
2	-ism	G	Suf.	病気・症状	病的状態(abnormal condition)	alcoholism(アルコール依存症)	alcohol「アルコール」
3	-itis	G	Suf.	病気・症状	〜炎(inflammation)	dermatitis(皮膚炎)	dermat(o)-「皮膚」
4	-lith	G	Suf.	病気・症状	石・結石(stone)	cystolith(膀胱結石)	cyst(o)-「膀胱」
5	-oma	G	Suf.	病気・症状	腫・瘤(tumor)	adenoma(腺腫)	aden(o)-「腺」
6	-osis	G	Suf.	病気・症状	病的状態(abnormal condition)	narcosis(昏睡状態)	narc(o)-「麻痺・麻酔・睡眠」
7	-agra	G	FCF	病気・症状	疼痛発作(sudden pain)	podagra(足部痛風)	pod(o)-「足」
8	-algia	G	FCF	病気・症状	〜痛(pain)	hepatalgia(肝臓痛)	hepat(o)-「肝臓」
9	-cele	G	FCF	病気・症状	腫瘍・ヘルニア(tumor / hernia)	hematocele(血瘤)	hemat(o)-「血」
10	-cephalus	G	FCF	病気・症状	頭部異常(abnormal condition of the head)	hydrocephalus(水頭症)	hydr(o)-「水」
11	-clasis	G	FCF	病気・症状	崩壊(breaking)	erythroclasis(赤血球崩壊)	erythr(o)-「赤・赤血球」
12	-emia / -aemia / -hemia / -haemia	G	FCF	病気・症状	〜な血液を有する状態(blood condition)	leukemia / leukaemia(白血病)	leuk(o)- / leuc(o)-「白・白血球」
13	-ia	G	FCF	病気・症状	病名をつくる(forming names of disorders)	leukemia / leukaemia(白血病)	ギリシャ・ラテン語系名詞接尾辞
14	-lexia	G	FCF	病気・症状	〜な(欠陥のある)読み方(condition of speech)	dyslexia(難読症)	dys-「困難な」
15	-mania	G	FCF	病気・症状	〜狂(extreme obsession)	mythomania(虚言症)	mytho-「神話」
16	-megaly	L	FCF	病気・症状	肥大(irregular enlargement)	cardiomegaly(心(臓)肥大(症))	cardi(o)-「心臓」
17	-odynia	G	FCF	病気・症状	〜痛(pain)	pododynia(足底痛)	pod(o)-「足」
18	-pathy	G	FCF	病気・症状	感情(feeling), 苦痛(suffering), 病気・〜症(disorder / disease), 療法(treatment)	neuropathy(神経障害), apathy(無感動・無関心)	neur(o)-「神経」, a-「無・不・非」
19	-penia	G	FCF	病気・症状	欠乏(deficiency)	sarcopenia(筋肉減少症)	sarc(o)-「肉」
20	-phagia / -phagy	G	FCF	病気・症状	食べること(eating)	dysphagia(嚥下障害)	dys-「困難な」
21	-phasia	G	FCF	病気・症状	言語障害(speech disorder)	dysphasia(不全失語症)	dys-「困難な」
22	-philia	G	FCF	病気・症状	〜の病的愛好(unnatural attraction)	pedophilia(小児性愛)	ped(o)- / paed(o)-「子供」
23	-phobia	G	FCF	病気・症状	恐怖症(extreme fear)	acrophobia(高所恐怖症)	acr(o)-「先端」
24	-phrenia	G	FCF	病気・症状	精神障害(mental disorder)	schizophrenia(統合失調症)	schiz-「分裂」
25	-phyte	G	FCF	病気・症状	増殖体(growth)	osteophyte(骨棘・骨増殖体)	oste(o)-「骨」
26	-plegia	G	FCF	病気・症状	麻痺(paralysis)	hemiplegia(半側麻痺)	hemi-「半」
27	-rrhage	G	FCF	病気・症状	異常流出(excessive and abnormal flow)	hemorrhage(大出血)	hem(o)-「血」
28	-rrhagia	G	FCF	病気・症状	異常流出(excessive and abnormal flow)	meningorrhagia(髄膜出血)	mening(o)-「髄膜」

(次ページに続く)

(表3のつづき)

	接辞と連結形	語源	接辞と連結形の分類	分野	意味(英語)	用例(日本語)	用例解説
29	-rrhea / -rrhoea	G	FCF	病気・症状	流出 (discharge / flow)	diarrhea(下痢)	dia-「～を通じて・～を横切って」
30	-rrhexis	G	FCF	病気・症状	破裂(rupture)	arteriorrhexis(動脈破裂)	arteri(o)-「動脈」
31	-schisis	G	FCF	病気・症状	亀裂(fissure)	palatoschisis(口蓋裂)	palato-「口蓋」
32	-tonia	L	FCF	病気・症状	緊張の状態 (condition of tention)	myotonia(筋緊張(症))	my(o)-「筋(肉)」
33	-uria	G	FCF	病気・症状	尿の状態 (urinary condition)	hematuria(血尿(症))	hemat(o)-「血」
34	-ics	G	Suf.	医学・医療・学問	～学(science), ～術(art)	orthopaedics / orthopedics(整形外科学)	orth(o)-「正しい」, p(a)ed(o)-「子供」
35	-acousia	G	FCF	医学・医療・学問	聴覚・聴取 (condition of hearing)	dysacousia(聴覚不全)	dys-「困難な」
36	-blast	G	FCF	医学・医療・学問	芽(sprout), 胚(embryo)	angioblast(血管芽細胞)	angi(o)-「血管」
37	-cide	L	FCF	医学・医療・学問	～を殺す薬剤 (agent that kills)	bactericide(殺菌剤)	bacteri-「細菌」
38	-cyte	G	FCF	医学・医療・学問	細胞(cell)	erythrocyte(赤血球)	erythr(o)-「赤・赤血球」
39	-derma	G	FCF	医学・医療・学問	皮膚(skin)	scleroderma(硬皮症)	scler(o)-「堅い」
40	-desis	G	FCF	医学・医療・学問	束縛・接合(binding together by surgery)	arthrodesis(関節固定(術))	arthr(o)-「関節」
41	-drome	G	FCF	医学・医療・学問	競走路(course), 走る(running)	syndrome(症候群)	syn-「同時に」
42	-ectomy	G	FCF	医学・医療・学問	切除(術)(excision)	gastrectomy(胃切除(術))	gastr(o)-「胃」
43	-gen	G	FCF	医学・医療・学問	～を生じるもの (a substance that produces something)	pathogen(病原菌・病原体)	path(o)-「病気, 苦痛」
44	-genesis	G	FCF	医学・医療・学問	発生・形成 (formation)	carcinogenesis(発癌)	carcin(o)-「癌」
45	-genic	G	FCF	医学・医療・学問	～を生み出す (producing)	carcinogenic(発癌性の)	carcin(o)-「癌」
46	-genous	G	FCF	医学・医療・学問	～を生み出す(producing), ～によって発生する(originating in)	myelogenous(骨髄性の)	myel(o)-「骨髄・脊髄」
47	-gnosia	G	FCF	医学・医療・学問	認識(recognition)	agnosia(失認)	a- / an-「不・無・非」
48	-gnosis	G	FCF	医学・医療・学問	認識(recognition)	prognosis(予後)	pro-「前」
49	-gram	G	FCF	医学・医療・学問	記録(record)	electrocardiogram(心電図)	electr(o)-「電気」, cardi(o)-「心臓」
50	-graph	G	FCF	医学・医療・学問	記録計器(instrument for recording)	electrocardiograph(心電計)	electr(o)-「電気」, cardi(o)-「心臓」
51	-graphy	G	FCF	医学・医療・学問	写法・記録法(process of recording)	electrocardiography(心電図記録法)	electr(o)-「電気」, cardi(o)-「心臓」
52	-iatrics	G	FCF	医学・医療・学問	医療・治療(medical treatment)	pediatrics / paediatrics(小児科学)	ped(o)- / paed(o)-「子供」
53	-iatry	G	FCF	医学・医療・学問	医療・治療(medical treatment)	psychiatry(精神医学)	psych(o)-「精神」
54	-kinesia	G	FCF	医学・医療・学問	運動(movement), 筋運動(muscular activity)	bradykinesia(動作緩慢)	brady-「遅い・緩慢な」
55	-kinesis	G	FCF	医学・医療・学問	運動(movement, activity)	chemokinesis(化学運動性)	chem(o)-「化学の」
56	-logist	G	FCF	医学・医療・学問	学者・専門家 (a person skilled in a branch of study)	ophthalmologist(眼科医)	ophthalm(o)-「目・眼」
57	-logy	G	FCF	医学・医療・学問	学問(study of)	cardiology(心臓(病)学)	cardi(o)-「心臓」

(次ページに続く)

（表3のつづき）

	接辞と連結形	語源	接辞と連結形の分類	分野	意味（英語）	用例（日本語）	用例解説
58	-lysis	G	FCF	医学・医療・学問	分解 (disintegration / decomposition)	analysis（分析）	ana-「上に」
59	-meter	G	FCF	医学・医療・学問	計器・〜計 (instrument for measuring)	goniometer（角度計）	goni(o)-「角」
60	-metry	G	FCF	医学・医療・学問	測定（法） (measurement)	craniometry（頭蓋計測法）	crani-「頭蓋（骨）」
61	-nomy	G	FCF	医学・医療・学問	知識体系 (system of knowledge regarding a field)	taxonomy（分類学）	tax(o)- / taxi-「順序・配列」
62	-opia	G	FCF	医学・医療・学問	視力障害 (visual disorder)	diplopia（複視・二重視）	dipl(o)-「複〜・二重〜」
63	-opsia / -opsy	G	FCF	医学・医療・学問	見ること (viewing)	myodesopsia（飛蚊症）, biopsy（生検）	*muioeides*「蚊のように（ギリシャ語）」+ -opsia, bi(o)-「生・生命・生物」
64	-orexia	G	FCF	医学・医療・学問	欲望 (desire), 食欲 (appetite)	anorexia（食欲不振・無食欲）, anorexia nervosa（神経性食欲不振・拒食症）	a- / an-「無・不・非」
65	-pepsia	G	FCF	医学・医療・学問	消化 (digestion)	dyspepsia（消化不良）	dys-「困難な」
66	-pexy	G	FCF	医学・医療・学問	固定 (surgical fixation)	enteropexy（腸固定術）	enter(o)-「腸」
67	-plasm	G	FCF	医学・医療・学問	形成するもの (formative substance)	cytoplasm（細胞質）	cyt(o)-「細胞」
68	-plasty	G	FCF	医学・医療・学問	形成（手術） (surgical repair)	mammoplasty / mammaplasty（乳房形成術）	mamm(o)- / mamma「乳房」
69	-pnea / -pnoea	G	FCF	医学・医療・学問	呼吸 (breathing)	hyperpnea / hyperpnoea（過呼吸）	hyper-「過度の」 cf. dyspnea, apnea, eupnea
70	-poiesis	G	FCF	医学・医療・学問	産出 (production), 形成 (formation)	hematopoiesis / hemopoiesis（造血・血液生成）	hemat(o)- / hem(o)-「血」
71	-praxia	G	FCF	医学・医療・学問	動作 (action)	apraxia（失行（症）・行動障害）	a- / an-「不・無・非」
72	-rrhaphy	G	FCF	医学・医療・学問	縫合 (suture)	enterorrhaphy（腸縫合術）	enter(o)-「腸」
73	-scope	G	FCF	医学・医療・学問	見る器械 (instrument to view)	endoscope（内視鏡）	end(o)-「内（部）」
74	-scopic	G	FCF	医学・医療・学問	観察の (pertaining to visual examination)	endoscopic（内視鏡検査の）	end(o)-「内（部）」
75	-scopy	G	FCF	医学・医療・学問	検査・観察 (process of visual examination)	endoscopy（内視鏡検査（法））	end(o)-「内（部）」
76	-stasis	G	FCF	医学・医療・学問	停止 (stopping)	homeostasis（恒常性）	home(o)-「類似の」
77	-stomy	G	FCF	医学・医療・学問	開口術 (forming a new opening)	gastrostomy（胃造瘻術）	gastr(o)-「胃」
78	-tome	G	FCF	医学・医療・学問	切断具 (instrument for cutting), 切片 (segment)	microtome（ミクロトーム）	micro-「小・微小」
79	-tomy	G	FCF	医学・医療・学問	切開（術） (cutting)	gastrotomy（胃切開（術））	gastr(o)-「胃」
80	-trophy	G	FCF	医学・医療・学問	栄養 (nourishment), 成長 (growth)	dystrophy（栄養障害・発育異常・筋萎縮）	dys-「困難な」
81	-iform / -form	L	FCF	大小・形・色・数量・状態・位置	〜の形を持つ (having the form of)	cuneiform（楔状骨の）	*cuneus*「楔（ラテン語）」
82	-able	L	Suf.	一般性が高い接尾辞	〜できる (can)	curable（治療できる）	*curabilis*（ラテン語，= cure + -able）より
83	-al	L	Suf.	一般性が高い接尾辞	〜に関する・〜の (relating to)	esophageal（食道の）	esophag(o)-「食道」
84	-ary	L	Suf.	一般性が高い接尾辞	〜に関する・〜の (pertaining to)	pulmonary（肺の）	pulmon(o)-「肺」
85	-cle / -cule	L	Suf.	一般性が高い接尾辞	小〜 (small)	saccule（小嚢）	ラテン語系名詞接尾辞

（次ページに続く）

(表3のつづき)

	接辞と連結形	語源	接辞と連結形の分類	分野	意味（英語）	用例（日本語）	用例解説
86	-er	OE	Suf.	一般性が高い接尾辞	〜する人（もの）(a person or thing that performs the action described by the verb)	helper（助手）	help「助ける」
87	-ician	F	Suf.	一般性が高い接尾辞	〜の専門家 (specialist)	pediatrician（小児科医）	pediatric「小児科の」
88	-ist	G	Suf.	一般性が高い接尾辞	〜の専門家 (specialist)	orthopaedist / orthopedist（整形外科医）	orth(o)-「正しい」, p(a)ed(o)-「子供」
89	-istic	G	Suf.	一般性が高い接尾辞	〜に関する・〜の (relating to)	linguistic（言語の）	lingu(o)-「言語・舌」
90	-ize / -ise	G	Suf.	一般性が高い接尾辞	〜化する (make / become)	minimize（最小にする）	minim(um)「最低限度」+ -ize
91	-oid	G	Suf.	一般性が高い接尾辞	〜に似た・〜のような (resembling / like)	arachnoid（クモ膜の）	arachn(o)-「クモ」
92	-ole	L	Suf.	一般性が高い接尾辞	小 (small)	arteriole（小動脈，細動脈）	arteri(o)-「動脈」
93	-or	L	Suf.	一般性が高い接尾辞	〜する人（もの）(a person or thing that performs the action described by the verb)	governor（統治者）	govern「統治する」

Index

欧文

abdominal　101
abdominal breathing　99
abdominal muscles　7
abnormal　104
acknowledge　19
activities of daily living（ADL）　7
acute pain　35
address　22
adjustment　62
adjustment disorder　59
advantageous　38
advise　67
aerobic exercise　15
affect　22
agnosia　79, 80
airway　102
akinesia　71, 72
alignment　30
alleviate　11
alveoli　103, 104
ambulation　6
amputate　59
angiostenosis　79, 80
annual　67
anterior　51
anterior spinal fusion（surgery）　52
anti-inflammatory　24
aphasia　79, 80
appropriate　67
approximately　54
apraxia　79, 80
arithmetic　107
arteriosclerosis　94, 96
artery　75
arthralgia　6, 8
arthritis　21
arthropathy　20, 21, 48
arthroplasty　16

articular　19
articular contracture　28
articular motion　20
assistive device　19
at one's earliest convenience　12
ataxia　79, 80
ataxic　111, 112
athetoid　111, 112
atrophy　45
atrophy of the multifidus muscles　44
attending physician　19
autoimmune　24
autonomous　62

be involved in　67
bedridden　6
bending position　44
bilateral　91
bony callus　28
bowlegged　11
bradykinesia　71, 72
break　27
brittle　38
Broca's area　76

carbohydrates　95
cardiovascular　38, 40
cartilage　14
cast　30
cauda equina　55
causative　62
caution　91
cerebral　75
cerebral palsy　107
cerebral sulcus　84
cerebral ventricle　84
cerebrovascular　38, 40
cerebrovascular disease　75

cervical 51, 53
characteristic 30
chief complaint 107
chronic 19
chronic lower back pain 43
chronic restrictive pulmonary disease（CRPD） 103
circumstance 88
clinical practice 107
Colles' fracture 27
comminuted fracture 31
competence 86
complication 94
comprehensive 22
conductor 67
conservative 14
contracture 54
contralateral 80
contribute 35
control 22
convalescent phase 79
COPD（chronic obstructive pulmonary disease） 99
coping skill 46
corticosteroids 23, 24
cough 99
cranial 78
crutch 110
cyst 15

daily chores 19
decline 86
deformation 110, 112
deformed 27
deformity 14
degenerative 14
degenerative disease 15
delivery 110
dementia 6, 8, 83
density 94
despite 83
deteriorate 83
deterioration 6
diabetes 35, 37
diabetes mellitus 91, 93
diabetic 91
diagnose 3, 21, 45

diagnosis 48
dialysis 94, 96
dietitian/dietician 104
diplegia 108, 109
disability 107
disease 69
dislocation 3
distal end of the radius/distal radius 28
disturb 99
dormitory 11
dorsal displacement of the fracture fragments 28
dorsiflexion 7, 8
dose 22
droop 70
dull 46
dysarthria 79, 80
dysesthesia/dysaesthesia 92, 93
dysfunction 24, 38
dysphagia 71, 72, 80
dystrophy 32

early detection 102
edema 30
elder-to-elder nursing 47
eliminate 59
empathize 51
encourage 35
endurance of the muscles 44
enthusiastic 11
Ewing's sarcoma 60
exacerbation 11
excessive 46
excessively 62
exercise tolerance 100
exhale 99, 101
exhausted 91
expansion 83
exposure 102
extension 27
external 30
external fixation 31

facility 67

Index **165**

fatal 110
femoral area 3
femoral head replacement 4
femoral neck fracture 3
femur 3
FEV1 100
fit 35
flaccid paraplegia 55
flex 27
flexibility 43
flexion 27
flexural 51
forearm 30
forward dislocation 51
fracture 3
fracture fragment 27
fracture line 28
full weight bearing 7
FVC 103

gangrene 94
gaze 59
genetics 14
glucose 94
goniometer 20, 21
grating sensation 15
grieve 59
groan 75
gymnasium 107

hamstring muscles 15
hand splints 23
health promotion 35
healthy life expectancy 38
hemiplegia 78, 80
hemisphere 75
hemorrhage/haemorrhage 78, 80
hemorrhagic 79
hesitate 35
hip abductor muscles 7
hip prosthesis 4
homeboundness 36
homemaker 19

hospitalization 75
hospitalize 3
hydrocephalus 84, 85
hyperglycemia 91, 93
hypoglycemic 94, 96

immobilize 30
immune 22
impress 107
inaccurately 83
inevitable 11
infarction 75
inflammation 102
inflammatory 19
inhale 99, 101
insomnia 62, 64
insulin preparation 95
intake 102
integral 75
intellectual 110
intensive 43
interfere 102
internal organ 38
internist 99
interphalangeal 29
interphalangeal joints 28
interprofessional 110, 112
intervention 86
intervertebral 40
intervertebral discs 39
intra-articular 32
intracerebral 78, 80
involuntary 70
irreversible 64
irritable 83
ischemic 78

junior 107
junior college 43

knee braces 15

knock knees 15

labor 110
labor of love 20
lap 59
lateral wedge insoles 15
left middle cerebral artery 76
linguistic 86, 88
locking plate 28
locomotive syndrome 35
locomotive system 38
loss of postural reflexes 71
lower extremity prosthesis 62
lower limb 6
lumbago 47, 48
lumbar 48
lumbar compression fracture 39
lumbar disc herniation 47
lumbar spinal canal stenosis 47
lumbosacral 56
lumbosacral spinal cord 55

manipulation 62
manipulative reduction 31
masking 71
maternity leave 43
medical records（chart） 107
medication 22
meniscus 15
metabolism 94
metacarpophalangeal 29
metacarpophalangeal joints 28
mild cognitive impairment 83
minimize 54, 69
mobility 6
mobility aids 23
mortality rate 78
motor paralysis 110
motor system 70
multiple 86
muscle tone（tonus） 108
muscular 6, 8

musculoskeletal ambulation disability symptom complex 39, 40
myodesopsia 93

necrosis 54
nephropathy 95, 96
neurology 85
neuropathy 95, 96
neurosurgery 75, 77
neurotransmission 54
neurotransmitter 70, 72
non-specific 47
nonsteroidal 24
nutritional 102

obesity 91
observe 70
obstruction 78
obstructive 99
obvious 86
ocular motility disorder 79
onset 14
open reduction and internal fixation 28
optimal treatment 23
optimistic 27
orally 75
orthopedic 3, 5, 45
orthopedist/orthopaedist 11, 21, 37
osteoarthritis 11, 13, 37
osteoarthritis of the knee 11
osteophyte 15, 16
osteoporosis 30, 32
overload 45
O 脚の bowlegged 11

palm 27
palmar flexion and ulnar deviation 31
pancreas 91
paralysis 54, 56
paraplegia 54, 56
Parkinson's disease 67

partial weight bearing　7
partition　59
pastime　35
pectoralis major　52
persistent　14
pharmacotherapy　62, 64
physical function　43
place emphasis on〜/place weight on〜　68
plantar flexion　7
pollution　102
post-menopausal　31, 32
postoperative　5, 6
postural　54
postural instability　71
posture　46
potent　22
pregnancy　110
prescribe　3, 16
prevalence　86
prior　30
prioritize　67
prognosis　24, 78
progressive　110
prospect　27
protocol　4
provision　46
pulmonary　75, 77
pulmonary aspiration　76
pulmonary rehabilitation　103
pursed-lip breathing　100

Q

quadriceps　15, 16
quadriplegia　51, 53

R

range of motion　6
reactive depression　63
ready-made　19
real feelings　68
recurrence　45
recurrence rate　43
reduction　31, 70
reflex sympathetic dystrophy　31
regenerative　51

reinforce　38
remission　23
renal failure　95
replacement arthroplasty　23
reposition　51
residual　86
resolve　46
respirator　54
respiratory　70
respite　83
resting tremor　71
restrictive ventilator impairment　108
retinopathy　91, 93
reunion　67
reveal　86
rheumatoid　21
rheumatoid arthritis　19
rib（thoracic）cage　100
rigidity　70

S

sarcoma　59, 61
scar formation　31
scoliosis　108, 109
secrete　91
secure　83
self-help device　51
senior　35
sensation　91
serratus anterior　52
share　43
shortness of breath　99
side effect　22
single-family house　4
sitting with two legs bent on each side　108
skull　78
smoking cessation clinic　99
spastic　111
special support school　108
specific lower back pain　47
spinal　40, 51
spinal canal stenosis　39, 48
spinal cord injury　51
spirometry　100, 101
splint　30
SpO_2　100

sputum 99
stabilize 54
stage 14
stenosis 40
stiffness 14
stimulus 86
stooped 70
strained back 46
strengthen 67
stressor 62
stroke 78
stump 59
stump plasty 60
subarachnoid 80
subarachnoid hemorrhage 79
subjective symptom 46
subsequent 43
substantia nigra 71
supervision 67, 69
supervisor 107
supine position 76
surface 27
surgical site 3
symmetrical 22
symptomatic depression 59

tenodesis 53
tenodesis-like action 52
tetraplegia 53
the Hoehn and Yahr scale 71
The Japanese Orthopedic Association 39
the neurology department 83
the perception of sensation in the plantar surface 7
therapeutic 14
therapeutic exercise 15
therapy 11
thigh 59
thoracic 56
thoracic cage ☞rib（thoracic）cage
thoracic cord injury 55

tibia 60
tomography 48
total knee arthroplasty（TKA） 15
toxic 102
transfer motion 7
transferring 43
tremendous 35
tremor 70
trigger 46
trunk expansion muscle 44

ulnar styloid 31
undergo 3
underlie 46
uneasy 83
urinary urgency and frequency 71
urine 94

vascular dementia 87
verbalize 62
vertebra 38
viscosity 94
vital capacity 102
vital prognoses 23
vital sign 59

walkable 11
waterproof 19
wear out 15
wheelchair 107
workload 43

X 脚 knock knees 15

和　文

あ

明らかな obvious　86
悪化 deterioration　☞低下，悪化 deterioration
（病気・症状の）悪化 exacerbation　11
扱い manipulation　☞操作，扱い manipulation
悪化させる deteriorate　83
アテトーゼ型の athetoid　111, 112
歩いて行ける walkable　11
安心な secure　83
安静時振戦 resting tremor　71
安定させる stabilize　54

い

息切れ shortness of breath　99
萎縮 atrophy　45
移乗，身体移動 transferring　43
移乗動作 transfer motion　7
異常な abnormal　104
一因となる contribute　35
1秒量 FEV1　100
一戸建て住宅 single-family house　4
遺伝（現象）genetics　14
移動補助具 mobility aids　23
医薬品，薬物 medication　22
インスリン製剤 insulin preparation　95

う

（治療などを）受ける undergo　☞（不愉快なことを）経験する，（治療などを）受ける undergo
うなる groan　75
運動器系 locomotive system　38
運動器不安定症 musculoskeletal ambulation disability symptom complex（MADS）　39
運動系 motor system　70
運動失調型の ataxic　111, 112
運動失調（症）ataxia　79, 80
運動耐用能 exercise tolerance　100
運動麻痺 motor paralysis　110
運動療法 therapeutic exercise　15

え

栄養士 dietitian/dietician　104
栄養に関する nutritional　102
栄養不良 dystrophy　☞発育異常，栄養不良，ジストロフィー dystrophy
壊死 necrosis　54
壊疽 gangrene　94
嚥下障害 dysphagia　71, 72, 80
炎症 inflammation　102
炎症性の，炎症を伴う inflammatory　19

お

（病気などが）（～を）冒す，襲う affect　22
怒りっぽい irritable　83
汚染 pollution　102
（病気などが）（～を）襲う affect　☞（病気などが）（～を）冒す，襲う affect
（～に）重きを置く，（～を）重視する place emphasis on～/place weight on～　68
およそ approximately　54

か

解決する resolve　46
外側楔状足底板 lateral wedge insoles　15
介入 intervention　86
回復期 convalescent phase　79
外部（から）の external　30
外面，表面 surface　27
拡大，膨張 expansion　83
角度計（ゴニオメーター）goniometer　20, 21
仮骨 bony callus　28
下肢 lower limb　6
過剰な excessive　46
過剰に excessively　62
形が崩れた deformed　☞変形した deformed
合併症 complication　94
可動域 range of motion　6
可動性 mobility　6
悲しむ grieve　59
仮面様顔貌 masking　71
カルテ medical records（chart）　107
寛解 remission　23
感覚，知覚 sensation　91

感覚異常 dysesthesia/dysaesthesia　92, 93
眼球運動障害 ocular motility disorder　79
環境，周囲の事情，境遇 circumstance　88
観血的整復固定術 open reduction and internal fixation　28
関節運動 articular motion　20
関節炎 arthritis　21
関節形成（術）arthroplasty　16
関節拘縮 articular contracture　28
関節症，関節疾患 arthropathy　20, 21, 48
関節置換術 replacement arthroplasty　23
関節痛 arthralgia　6, 8
関節内の intra-articular　32
関節の articular　19
関節リウマチ rheumatoid arthritis　19
（〜を）感動させる impress　107
監督，管理 supervision　67, 69
緩和する alleviate　☞軽減する，緩和する alleviate

奇形 deformity　14
きしむような感じ grating sensation　15
寄宿舎，寮 dormitory　11
既製品の ready-made　19
義足 lower extremity prosthesis　62
基礎となる underlie　46
きっかけとなる trigger　46
（観察によって）気づく observe　☞（観察によって）認める，気づく observe
ぎっくり腰 strained back　46
気道 airway　102
機能障害 dysfunction　24, 38
気晴らし pastime　35
ギプス（包帯）cast　30
休息 respite　83
胸郭 rib（thoracic）cage　100
強化する reinforce　38
共感する empathize　51
境遇 circumstance　☞環境，周囲の事情，境遇 circumstance
狭窄症 stenosis　40
胸髄損傷 thoracic cord injury　55
胸部の thoracic　56
虚血性の ischemic　78
禁煙外来 smoking cessation clinic　99
筋緊張 muscle tone（tonus）　108

筋持久力 endurance of the muscles　44
筋の muscular　6, 8

口すぼめ呼吸 pursed-lip breathing　100
屈曲 flexion　27
屈曲の flexural　51
くも膜下出血 subarachnoid hemorrhage　79
くも膜下の subarachnoid　80
車椅子 wheelchair　107

け

（患者の治療を実行するための）計画 protocol　4
（不愉快なことを）経験する，（治療などを）受ける undergo　3
軽減する，緩和する alleviate　11
警告する caution　91
脛骨 tibia　60
痙直型の spastic　111
頸椎固定手術 anterior spinal fusion（surgery）　52
経度認知障害 mild cognitive impairment　83
頸部の cervical　51, 53
激痛 acute pain　35
血管狭窄 angiostenosis　79, 80
血糖降下の hypoglycemic　☞低血糖（症）の hypoglycemic
原因となる causative　62
健康寿命 healthy life expectancy　38
健康増進 health promotion　35
健康な fit　35
腱固定 tenodesis　53
腱固定作用 tenodesis-like action　52
言語の linguistic　86, 88
減少 reduction　70

抗炎症（性）の anti-inflammatory　24
構音障害 dysarthria　79, 80
高血糖 hyperglycemia　91, 93
拘縮 contracture　54
梗塞 infarction　75
拘束性喚起障害 restrictive ventilator impairment　108

口頭で orally　75

効力のある，よく効く potent　22
誤嚥 pulmonary aspiration　76
股関節外転筋 hip abductor muscles　7
呼吸器の respiratory　70
呼吸リハビリテーション pulmonary rehabilitation
　　103
黒質 substantia nigra　71
腰の lumbar　48
固縮 rigidity　70
骨格筋の musculoskeletal ambulation disability
　　symptom complex　40
骨関節炎 osteoarthritis　11, 13, 37
骨棘，骨増殖体 osteophyte　15, 16
骨折線 fracture line　28
骨折 fracture　3
骨増殖体 osteophyte　☞骨棘，骨増殖体 osteophyte
骨粗鬆症 osteoporosis　30, 32
骨片 fracture fragment　27
骨片の手背側へのずれ dorsal displacement of the
　　fracture fragments　28
固定する immobilize　30
言葉で表す verbalize　62
ゴニオメーター goniometer　☞角度計（ゴニオメー
　　ター）goniometer
娯楽，気晴らし pastime　35
コルチコステロイド corticosteroids　23, 24
コレス骨折 Colles' fracture　27
こわばり stiffness　14

最小限にする，最小にする minimize　54, 69
再生の regenerative　51
最適治療 optimal treatment　23
再発 recurrence　45
再発率 recurrence rate　43
避けられない，不可避の inevitable　11
下げる droop　☞垂れる，下げる droop
左中大脳動脈 left middle cerebral artery　76
さらすこと exposure　102
（活動などに）参加する，携わる be involved in　67
産休 maternity leave　43
算数 arithmetic　107
残存の residual　86

自覚症状 subjective symptom　46
弛緩性対麻痺 flaccid paraplegia　55
指揮者 conductor　67
仕切る partition　59
刺激 stimulus　86
仕事量 workload　43
自己免疫（性）autoimmune　24
四肢麻痺 quadriplegia/tetraplegia　51, 53
自助具 self-help device　51
ジストロフィー dystrophy　☞発育異常，栄養不良，
　　ジストロフィー dystrophy
姿勢 posture　46
姿勢の postural　☞体位の，姿勢の postural
姿勢反射障害（姿勢の不安定）postural instability
　　71
姿勢反射の喪失 loss of postural reflexes　71
施設，設備 facility　67
指節間関節 interphalangeal joints　28
指節間の interphalangeal　29
持続性の persistent　14
失語（症）aphasia　79, 80
失行（症）apraxia　79, 80
失動 akinesia　☞無動，失動 akinesia
失認（症）agnosia　79, 80
疾病，疾患 disease　☞病気，疾病，疾患 disease
指導教官 supervisor　107
四頭筋 quadriceps　15, 16
死亡率 mortality rate　78
示す，見せる reveal　86
尺骨茎状突起 ulnar styloid　31
（～を）重視する place emphasis on～/place weight
　　on～　☞（～に）重きを置く，（～を）重視する
　　place emphasis on～/place weight on～
集中的な intensive　43
柔軟性 flexibility　43
主治医（担当医）attending physician　19
手術後の postoperative　5, 6
手術部位 surgical site　3
主訴 chief complaint　107
手装具 hand splints　23
（大量の）出血 hemorrhage/haemorrhage　78, 80
出血性 hemorrhagic　79
出産 delivery　110
主婦 homemaker　19

障がい disability　107
衝撃を弱める break　27
症候性うつ状態 symptomatic depression　59
掌尺屈位 palmar flexion and ulnar deviation　31
承認する acknowledge　19
除去する eliminate　59
助言する advise　67
処方する prescribe　3, 16
自律した autonomous　62
神経学 neurology　85
（脳）神経外科（学）neurosurgery　75, 77
神経障害 neuropathy　95, 96
神経伝達 neurotransmission　54
神経伝達物質 neurotransmitter　70, 72
神経内科 the neurology department　83
人工股関節 hip prosthesis　4
人工呼吸装置 respirator　54
人工骨頭置換術 femoral head replacement　4
人工膝関節全置換術 total knee arthroplasty（TKA）　15
進行性の progressive　110
真正糖尿病 diabetes mellitus　93
振戦，震え tremor　70
心臓血管の cardiovascular　38, 40
腎臓病 nephropathy　95, 96
身体移動 transferring　☞移乗，身体移動 transferring
身体機能 physical function　43
診断 diagnosis　48
診断する diagnose　3, 21, 45
伸展 extension　27
腎不全 renal failure　95

吸い込む inhale　99, 101
膵臓 pancreas　91
水頭症 hydrocephalus　84, 85
頭蓋骨 skull　78
頭蓋の，頭部の cranial　78
好きでする仕事 labor of love　20
ストレスを引き起こす要因 stressor　62
擦り減る wear out　15

整形外科医 orthopedist/orthopaedist　11, 21, 37
整形外科の orthopedic　3, 5, 45
整復 reduction　31
整復させる reposition　51
生命徴候 vital sign　59
生命予後 vital prognoses　23
咳 cough　99
脊髄損傷 spinal cord injury　51
脊髄の spinal　51
脊柱管狭窄症 spinal canal stenosis　39, 48
脊柱側弯（症）scoliosis　108, 109
脊柱の spinal　40
摂取 intake　102
切断する amputate　59
設備 facility　☞施設，設備 facility
全荷重 full weight bearing　7
前鋸筋 serratus anterior　52
前屈姿勢 bending position　44
前方脱臼 forward dislocation　51
専門職間の interprofessional　110, 112
前腕 forearm　30

創外固定 external fixation　31
早期発見 early detection　102
操作，扱い manipulation　62
添え木，副子 splint　30
足底の感覚（知覚）the perception of sensation in the plantar surface　7
その後の subsequent　43

体育館 gymnasium　107
体位の，姿勢の postural　54
対応能力 coping skill　46
大学3年生 junior　107
大学4年生 senior　35
体幹伸展筋 trunk expansion muscle　44
大胸筋 pectoralis major　52
退行性の degenerative　☞変性の，退行性の degenerative
代謝 metabolism　94
対称性の symmetrical　22
（〜に）対処する address　22
大腿 thigh　59
大腿骨 femur　3

Index **173**

大腿骨頸部骨折 femoral neck fracture　3
大腿部 femoral area　3
大脳の cerebral　☞脳の，大脳の cerebral
（活動などに）携わる be involved in　☞（活動などに）参加する，携わる be involved in
多大な，途方もなく大きい tremendous　35
脱臼 dislocation　3
ためらう hesitate　35
多裂筋の萎縮 atrophy of the multifidus muscles　44
垂れる，下げる droop　70
痰 sputum　99
段階 stage　14
炭水化物 carbohydrates　95
断層撮影 tomography　48
短大 junior college　43
断端，付け根 stump　59
断端形成 stump plasty　60
担当医 attending physician　19

知覚 sensation　☞感覚，知覚 sensation
致命的な fatal　110
注視 gaze　59
中手指節関節 metacarpophalangeal joints　28
中手指節の metacarpophalangeal　29
治療（上）の therapeutic　14
治療，療法 therapy　11
知力（知能）の intellectual　110

つ

椎間の intervertebral　40
椎間板 intervertebral discs　39
椎間板ヘルニア lumbar disc herniation　47
椎骨 vertebra　38
対麻痺 paraplegia　54, 56
疲れ果てた exhausted　91
都合がつき次第 at one's earliest convenience　☞できるだけ早く，都合がつき次第 at one's earliest convenience
（～を）強める strengthen　67

低下 decline　86
低下，悪化 deterioration　6

提供 provision　46
底屈 plantar flexion　7
低血糖（症）の hypoglycemic　94, 96
適応 adjustment　62
適応障害 adjustment disorder　59
適切な appropriate　67
できるだけ早く，都合がつき次第 at one's earliest convenience　12
掌，手のひら palm　27

橈骨遠位端 distal end of the radius/distal radius　28
動作緩慢 bradykinesia　71, 72
透析 dialysis　94, 96
同窓会，懇親会 reunion　67
糖尿病 diabetes　35, 37
糖尿病 diabetes mellitus　91
糖尿病患者 diabetic　91
頭部に近い anterior　☞前の，頭部に近い anterior
頭部の cranial　78
動脈 artery　75
動脈血酸素飽和度 SpO_2　100
動脈硬化（症）arteriosclerosis　94, 96
投与量 dose　☞服用量，投与量 dose
特異的腰痛 specific lower back pain　47
特別支援学校 special support school　108
特有な characteristic　30
（高齢者の）閉じこもり homeboundness　36
徒手整復 manipulative reduction　31
途方もなく大きい tremendous　☞多大な，途方もなく大きい tremendous
努力肺活量 FVC　103

内科医 internist　99
内臓 internal organ　38
軟骨 cartilage　14

肉腫 sarcoma　59, 61
日常生活活動（ADL）activities of daily living　7
日常の仕事 daily chores　19
（痛みが）鈍い dull　46

日本整形外科学会 The Japanese Orthopedic
　　Association　39
〜にもかかわらず despite　83
入院 hospitalization　75
（〜を）入院させる hospitalize　3
尿 urine　94
尿意逼迫と頻尿 urinary urgency and frequency　71
妊娠 pregnancy　110
認知症 dementia　6, 8, 83

寝たきりの bedridden　6
熱心な enthusiastic　11
粘性 viscosity　94

の

脳血管障害 cerebrovascular disease　75
脳血管性認知症 vascular dementia　87
脳血管の cerebrovascular　38, 40
脳溝 cerebral sulcus　84
脳室 cerebral ventricle　84
（脳）神経外科（学）neurosurgery　75, 77
脳性麻痺 cerebral palsy　107
脳卒中 stroke　78
濃度 density　94
脳内の intracerebral　78, 80
脳の，大脳の cerebral　75
嚢胞 cyst　15
能力 competence　86

は

背臥位 supine position　76
肺活量 vital capacity　102
肺活量測定 spirometry　100, 101
背屈 dorsiflexion　7, 8
配置 alignment　30
肺の pulmonary　75, 77
肺胞 alveoli　103, 104
（息を）吐き出す exhale　99, 101
パーキンソン病 Parkinson's disease　67
（〜するように）働きかける，励ます encourage　35
発育異常，栄養不良，ジストロフィー dystrophy
　　　32
（病気などの）発病，発症 onset　14

馬尾神経 cauda equina　55
ハムストリングス hamstring muscles　15
半球 hemisphere　75
半月板 meniscus　15
瘢痕形成 scar formation　31
反射性交感神経ジストロフィー reflex sympathetic
　　dystrophy　31
（体の）反対側の contralateral　80
反応性うつ reactive depression　63

ひざ（座ったときの下腹部からひざ頭までの部分）
　　lap　59
膝装具 knee braces　15
非ステロイド性の nonsteroidal　24
必須の integral　☞不可欠な，必須の integral
非特異的 non-specific　47
飛蚊症 myodesopsia　93
肥満 obesity　91
病気，疾病，疾患 disease　69
表面 surface　☞外面，表面 surface

不安な uneasy　83
不可逆的な irreversible　64
不可欠な，必須の integral　75
不可避の inevitable　☞避けられない，不可避の
　　inevitable
副作用 side effect　22
副子 splint　☞添え木，副子 splint
腹式呼吸 abdominal breathing　99
複数の multiple　86
腹部の abdominal　101
服用量，投与量 dose　22
浮腫 edema　30
不随意の，意思によらない involuntary　70
不正確に inaccurately　83
負担をかけすぎる overload　45
腹筋 abdominal muscles　7
ブドウ糖 glucose　94
部分荷重 partial weight bearing　7
不眠（症）insomnia　62, 64
震え tremor　☞振戦，震え tremor
ブローカ野 Broca's area　76

プロトコル，（患者の治療を実行するための）計画 protocol　4
粉砕骨折 comminuted fracture　31
分担する share　43
分泌する secrete　91
分娩の過程 labor　110

閉経後の post-menopausal　31, 32
閉塞 obstruction　78
閉塞性の obstructive　99
変形 deformation　110, 112
変形，奇形 deformity　14
変形した deformed　27
変形性関節症（骨関節炎）osteoarthritis　11, 13, 37
変形性膝関節症 osteoarthritis of the knee　11
変性疾患 degenerative disease　15
変性の，退行性の degenerative　14
片麻痺 hemiplegia　78, 80

妨害する disturb　99
妨害する interfere　102
包括的な comprehensive　22
防水の waterproof　19
膨張 expansion　☞拡大，膨張 expansion
ホーエン・ヤールの重症度分類 the Hoehn and Yahr scale　71
歩行 ambulation　6
保存的な conservative　14
補助器具 assistive device　19

ま

毎年の annual　☞例年の，毎年の annual
前かがみの stooped　70
前の，頭部に近い anterior　51
前の prior　30
（関節を）曲げる flex　27
松葉づえ crutch　110
麻痺 paralysis　54, 56
慢性拘束性肺疾患 chronic restrictive pulmonary disease　103
慢性の chronic　19

慢性閉塞性肺疾患 COPD（chronic obstructive pulmonary disease）　99
慢性腰痛症 chronic lower back pain　43

見込み prospect　☞見通し，予想，見込み prospect
見せる reveal　☞示す，見せる reveal
見通し，予想，見込み prospect　27
（観察によって）認める，気づく observe　70

無動，失動 akinesia　71, 72

免疫 immune　22

網膜症 retinopathy　91, 93
もろい brittle　38

薬物 medication　☞医薬品，薬物 medication
薬物療法 pharmacotherapy　62, 64

ゆ

ユーイング肉腫 Ewing's sarcoma　60
有益な advantageous　38
有酸素運動 aerobic exercise　15
（〜を）優先させる prioritize　67
有毒な toxic　102
有病率 revalence　86

腰仙髄 lumbosacral spinal cord　55
腰仙の lumbosacral　56
腰椎圧迫骨折 lumbar compression fracture　39
腰痛 lumbago　47, 48
腰部脊柱管狭窄症 lumbar spinal canal stenosis　47
抑制する control　22
予後 prognosis　24, 78

予想 prospect　☞見通し，予想，見込み prospect

楽天的な optimistic　27

リウマチ性 rheumatoid　21
寮 dormitory　☞寄宿舎，寮 dormitory
両側の bilateral　91
療法 therapy　☞治療，療法 therapy
両麻痺 diplegia　108, 109
臨床実習 clinical practice　107

例年の，毎年の annual　67

老老介護 elder-to-elder nursing　47
ロコモティブシンドローム locomotive syndrome　35
ロッキング・プレート locking plate　28

わ

割り座 sitting with two legs bent on each side　108

シンプル理学療法学・作業療法学シリーズ
リハビリテーション英語テキスト

2017年2月20日　第1刷発行	監修者　細田多穂
2020年2月20日　第2刷発行	編集者　飯島博之，濱口豊太，隈元庸夫
2022年2月10日　第3刷発行	発行者　小立健太

発行所　株式会社　南　江　堂
〒113-8410　東京都文京区本郷三丁目42番6号
☎(出版)03-3811-7235　(営業)03-3811-7239
ホームページ https://www.nankodo.co.jp/
印刷　三報社印刷／製本　ブックアート
装丁　node（野村里香）

English for Students of Rehabilitation
© Nankodo Co., Ltd., 2017

定価は表紙に表示してあります．
落丁・乱丁の場合はお取り替えいたします．
ご意見・お問い合わせはホームページまでお寄せ下さい．

Printed and Bound in Japan
ISBN 978-4-524-25719-5

本書の無断複写を禁じます．
JCOPY〈出版者著作権管理機構　委託出版物〉
本書の無断複写は，著作権法上での例外を除き，禁じられています．複写される場合は，そのつど事前に，出版者著作権管理機構（TEL 03-5244-5088，FAX 03-5244-5089，e-mail: info@jcopy.or.jp）の許諾を得てください．

本書をスキャン，デジタルデータ化するなどの複製を無許諾で行う行為は，著作権法上での限られた例外（「私的使用のための複製」など）を除き禁じられています．大学，病院，企業などにおいて，内部的に業務上使用する目的で上記の行為を行うことは私的使用には該当せず違法です．また私的使用のためであっても，代行業者等の第三者に依頼して上記の行為を行うことは違法です．